Hoxsey

When Natural Cures for Cancer Became Illegal

The Historical Autobiography of Harry Hoxsey, N.D.

You Don't Have to Die
reprinted by
Transpersonal Publishing

For additional copies, retail, or wholesale quantities of this book, or
other related books or CDs, contact the publisher:

Transpersonal Publishing
div. AHU, LLC
PO Box 7220
Kill Devil Hills, NC 27948
800-296-MIND
www.TranspersonalPublishing.com

Distributed by SCB Distributors
Available through all major wholesalers in North America

Note: New Authors- We do not handle any queries over the phone;
see submission guidelines on our website.

Text is FSC recycled paper, representative of the cover symbols

Manufactured in the United States of America by TPS

This book is humbly dedicated to Martha B. Hoxsey, who endowed me with the flesh and bone and blood to endure the struggle; to Dr. John C. Hoxsey, who taught me to love suffering humanity and minister to its ills, and thus inspired the struggle; to Martha H., "Skipper" and "Patty" Hoxsey, who are the main incentive to keep on pitching 'til I win.

TABLE OF CONTENTS

"There is a principle which is a bar against all information, which is proof against all argument, and which cannot fail to keep a man in everlasting ignorance. That principle is condemnation without investigation."

HERBERT SPENCER

Introduction

This is a fascinating, historical account of how Harry Hoxsey, ND, single-handedly fought the American Medical Association (AMA) on the efficacy of Hoxsey Therapy (an herbal, all-natural cancer therapy) and won...proving, at that time, "Hoxsey Therapy" was an effective treatment against cancer. It was only a few weeks later, however, when the seventeen Hoxsey clinics established throughout the United States were pad-locked by the Food and Drug Administration (FDA). Shortly thereafter, the headquarters in Dallas, TX, moved to Tijuana, Mexico, where they continued to operate as the BioMedical Center (BMC). Although "integrative medicine" (combining conventional and natural medicines) tends to be a common choice for cancer patients today, there are many cancer patients who have been given up on by conventional medicine who turn to Hoxsey Therapy, just as in Dr. Hoxsey's day.

After this book was published, several anecdotal studies had been conducted by credible sources, including the National Institutes of Health (NIH) department of alternative and complementary medicine, which showed a significant number of patients surviving many years after turning to Hoxsey Therapy as a last resort. Also, after visiting the clinic, I met patients with friends and family members who have experienced long-term survival rates, and therefore many of them use Hoxsey Therapy as a first line of defense against cancer and other autoimmune diseases.

It may be fair to say that today the AMA takes a "hands-off" approach to integrative medicine, particularly after the NIH began researching natural remedies for cancer and congress passed a law giving the public the right to choose alternative medicines in the latter part of the 20th century. However, the FDA continues to scrutinize the labels of natural cancer remedies; and perhaps in many cases rightfully so, as some may simply attempt to cash-in on the multi-billion dollar industry of cancer therapy with unfounded claims and inept research.

Nonetheless, this book has impressive history worth considering when eclectic physicians, or "naturopathic doctors" as we refer to today, fought advocates for conventional medicine in a showdown to prove the efficacy of natural medicine in the treatment of cancer. Harry Hoxsey eventually won his case by proving Hoxsey Therapy cured external cancers, reflected in several case histories in this book. While Hoxsey Therapy continues to maintain a good track record in many regards, it is still illegal to label it as a cancer treatment or remedy. In the end, it is the patient's responsibility to use discernment when considering his or her right to choose a complementary or alternative approach.

Allen Chips, DCH, PhD, Author
Killing Your Cancer Without Killing Yourself: Using Natural Cures That Work (First Edition, 2006)
Killing Your Cancer: With Natural, Alternative, and Complementary Medicines (Revised Second Edition, 2010)

CHAPTER ONE

They Don't Want to Die

Suppose you suddenly discovered that you have cancer. A horrible, crab-like disease has invaded your body, is gnawing your flesh, has pushed greedy tentacles into your vital organs. A loathsome scavenger slowly and inexorably is consuming you alive, cell by cell.

The doctor says it's too far advanced for treatment. As gently as anyone ever pronounced a death sentence on another human being, he tells you: "You may live a year, you may die in six months." Nothing on earth can save you, medical science can do little more than ease the excruciating physical pain that inevitably accompanies later stages of this dread disease.

You stumble home, numbly set about putting your affairs in order. You make a will. You assemble the documents relating to your "estate"—insurance policies, the deed to the house, title to the car and other personal property—and put them in a safe place where your family can find them after you're "gone."

Your mind recoils in horror. You don't want to die.

During the ensuing weeks the hopeless anguish of members of your family is only too apparent beneath the thin veneer of cheery solicitude. They tiptoe past your door as past the coffin of the dead. The hushed voices and funereal smiles of friends and relatives who drop in reveal only too clearly that they, too, already have mentally con-

1

signed you to the grave. Everywhere you turn you are confronted by signs that your impending doom is an accepted fact.

But your heart still beats, the blood pulses in your veins, your lungs inhale and exhale air, you're still alive! And you don't want to die!

Then one day a friend brings you a magazine with an article about a man who claims that he has a treatment that cures cancer. Not all cases, but a goodly percentage. And he allegedly has cured many patients who originally were given up as incurable by their own doctors.

With a faint spark of hope you read avidly. You learn that this healer is not an M.D., that the American Medical Association has denounced him as a "quack" and says the medicine that is the basis of his unorthodox treatment (he uses no surgery, x-ray or radium) is little more potent than cough syrup. You are surprised to discover that the AMA has never actually tested his treatment although the healer repeatedly has begged for such an investigation, although hundreds of his patients have testified this treatment saved their lives, although several courts have held that it actually cures cancer.

The case histories of a few patients at his clinic are detailed in the magazine, and you read them with tense interest. Most of these people seem to have been in just as critical a condition as you when they started this treatment. Yet they apparently recovered, and years later they are still alive. Their accounts are very convincing.

By the time you reach the end of the article the spark of hope within you has been fanned into bright flame. If these stories are true, if this treatment actually cured these cancer victims, perhaps it can do the same for you!

You get in touch with your doctor, show him the article. He glances at it, tosses it down and dismisses it with one word: "Rubbish!" He tells you that there is no known chemical cure for cancer, that this alleged healer is a notorious quack; if you go to him, all you'll do is waste your time and money.

Time and money mean nothing to a dead man, you grimly remind him. Does he have anything better to offer?

He shakes his head. Perhaps x-ray or radium would help to buy you a little breathing space. But to be brutally frank, your case is hopeless, nothing short of a miracle will save you. . . .

What would you do?

Would you remain at home, praying for death to relieve you from pain and suffering? Or would you immediately set out for the clinic of this unorthodox healer who at the very least offers you a chance to fight for your life?

During the past 33 years at least 20,000 cancer victims in this country have faced this problem, and chosen the second course of action. They came to me with the same pathetic plea: "I don't want to die. Save me!" We've never turned any of them away, providing there was even an outside chance that my treatment would help them.

We're not miracle men, we don't profess to cure all cases of cancer, we don't guarantee a cure. Nevertheless thousands of men, women and children once stricken with cancer are still alive today as the result of our treatment.

I defy any other doctor or hospital on earth to match that record.

When I first came to grips with cancer, in the 1920s, it was just another disease. The medical spotlight was on tuberculosis, at that time the nation's No. 2 killer, and on venereal diseases. Since then science, with the aid of "miracle drugs," has effectively conquered both these plagues. Unfortunately it has proven an absolute flop in its efforts to cope with, or even to contain, the third and deadliest plague afflicting mankind.

Look at the statistics.

During the past 30 years the number of cancer deaths has more than doubled in nearly every civilized nation on the globe. It is estimated that between 3 and 4 million people contract this disease every year. Every 10 seconds someone, somewhere on earth, dies of cancer. That makes 360 deaths per hour, 8,640 per day, more than 3 million deaths every year!

No pestilence known to history has taken such a fearful toll of human life. The awful cycle of epidemics known as the "Black Death" that practically depopulated Europe during the dark 14th century is estimated to have carried off a total of 25 million victims. Today in the 20th century, despite our vaunted advance in medical knowledge and all the miracles of modern science, cancer snuffs out more lives every decade than the "Black Death" did in its entire 100-year reign of terror!

In the U.S. about 250,000 people die of this dread disease every year. Except for the various diseases of the heart, no other scourge claims as many victims among our people. Cancer now causes 5 times as many deaths as influenza and pneumonia combined, 10 times as many as tuberculosis, 80 times as many as polio. And the shocking mortality rate keeps right on rising, with an average increase of 5,000 more cancer deaths each succeeding year.

Cancer is more devastating than war. Every year it takes twice as many American lives as were lost on all the battlefields of World War I, half as many as were lost in World War II, ten times as many as in the Korean War.

It is more costly than accidents of all types. Every year it causes 6 times as many deaths as automobiles do, 4 times as many as all other accidents combined.

It is deadlier than the atom bomb. Every year it kills twice as many people in this country as died in the A-bombing of both Hiroshima and Nagasaki.

It stalks every man, woman and child in the land. The National Cancer Institute estimates that 50 million people now living in this country—nearly one out of every three —eventually will contract cancer; that at least 25 million of them—nearly one-sixth our present total population —eventually will die of this terrible disease.

Imagine for a moment that a virulent plague wiped out the entire population of Miami, Florida last year. This year it destroys all life in Omaha, Nebraska. Next year it will erase Akron, Ohio from the map. Every 12 months it converts another major American city into a vast cemetery.

That, in effect, is what cancer is now doing to this country.

What hope can medical science offer us?

At this writing organized medicine recognizes only two types of treatment for cancer; surgery and irradiation (x-ray, radium or radioactive isotopes). The number of actual cures achieved by these authorized methods remains pitifully few. Of victims treated in the primary stage of the disease, it recently was admitted, only 55 or

56 percent survive; of those who reach the fourth stage, none survive.

These scandalous figures highlight the tragic failure of modern medicine to measure up to the deadliest plague of our times. But no statistics, however sensational, are eloquent enough to portray the horror, terror, physical suffering and mental anguish of the victim and his family, nor the corroding despair that accompanies his frantic search for a reprieve from death.

No other disease arouses such direct and universal fear in mankind. In the mind of the public, a diagnosis of cancer is the equivalent of a death sentence. Current hysteria at the mere mention of the word "cancer" is such that most doctors will not hand the verdict to the victim himself; they confide it to members of his family. And children let beloved parents die, husbands let their wives die, rather than reveal the awful, shameful secret.

Seldom a day passes in our clinic without a long distance telephone call from some part of the country: "Can you treat my father (mother, brother, sister, wife or husband) without letting him know he has cancer?"

That of course is impossible; just because an individual is sick, he isn't necessarily a moron.

"He'll kill himself, if he finds out!"

In vain we point out that very few cancer patients ever commit suicide, especially if given a chance to fight for their lives.

But reason seldom prevails in an atmosphere poisoned by irrational terror. They prefer to let their loved ones "die in peace"—and ignorance.

Doctors themselves are often infected by panic. They have little confidence in the treatments they perforce prescribe; experience has taught them that few patients stricken with the dread disease survive long. Today, when the average physician discovers that his patient has cancer, even before he opens his mouth to deliver the diagnosis he has given up hope, mentally consigned the helpless wretch to death. If he is frank, he will tell the victim (or relatives) that the latter has three months, perhaps six months, perhaps a year to live.

Their hopelessness is contagious. Uusually, sometime within the prescribed period or shortly thereafter, the doomed individual obediently lies down and dies.

I contend that a great many of these deaths are unnecessary. Many of these unfortunates do not die of cancer. In the final analysis, they are frightened to death!

No case of cancer, however far advanced, is entirely hopeless. Thousands of cancer victims who were told by doctors that they would die within six or eight months are still alive and healthy years later, and now show no trace of the dread disease!

The fact that we cure cancer without the use of surgery, x-ray or radium has been established in open court on numerous occasions by the testimony of hundreds of recovered patients. The witnesses exhibit photos showing hideous growths on various parts of the body, give harrowing accounts of long and ineffective treatment by conventional methods before they came to our clinic. And they show clean scar tissue where the cancer fell away "like the pit from a peach" after a few months of our treatment. Others, internal cases, tell how they came to the Hoxsey clinic after their physicians gave them up as incurable and sent them home to die, how they live on to confound their doctors.

Did these people actually have cancer? We produce records showing diagnosis by their own doctors, and biopsy reports from leading pathological laboratories.

Are they really cured? The average life of a cancer victim is about two years after the onset of the disease. The witnesses were treated 5, 10, in some instances 20 years ago, and they are still alive, free of any trace of the disease.

Such overwhelming evidence has convinced judges, juries, U.S. Senators, Federal and State investigating committees, as well as numerous doctors that we cure cancer. The refusal of organized medicine to recognize or even investigate my treatment will be dealt with in detail in future chapters. In part, this opposition stems from the fact that I am not an M.D. (although I employ qualified and licensed practitioners at my clinic). Yet the celebrated scientist Alexis Carrel has declared:

> "More than half the great remedies known to medical history have come from empiricists; that is from 'irregulars,' men and women of no or little scientific training. There is no reason to believe that conditions have essentially changed. In the future an unregistered, self-trained experimenter, an 'empiricist' by strict classification, may just as well make a revolutionary medical discovery as one employed in a great laboratory having every up-to-date equipment."

So I am an "empiricist." My treatment is based on experience and practice.

Today the Hoxsey Clinic at Dallas, Texas is the largest independent cancer clinic in the world, with some 10,000 cases under constant treatment or observation. And day by day more patients stream in from every section of the

United States, Canada and Mexico. They come by bus, train, plane and private auto; some hobble in on crutches, others are brought in on litters or in wheel chairs.

What kind of people are they? What drives them to our clinic for treatment, frequently against the advice of trusted family physicians?

If you were to come to our clinic, sit in a waiting room and talk with some of our patients, here are a few of the stories you'd hear:

No. 1—This elderly man sat in a trailer camp in Arizona a few days ago, contemplating suicide. He has cancer of the prostate and the doctors say it is incurable. A carpenter by trade, he can no longer work; his wife has had to take a job in a laundry to support them. Having seen his father and brother die of the same disease, he had no desire to prolong his agony. So he sat there, a loaded revolver on the table, trying to nerve himself to the deed. At that moment there was a knock on the door and a neighbor came in with an account of the Hoxsey treatment. He immediately phoned his wife, told her to quit her job. That same night they hitched up their trailer and set off for Dallas.

No. 2—The parchment-faced young man in a wheel chair says he is from California. Doctors there performed an exploratory operation, discovered his intestines were riddled with cancer, decided he is inoperable, sewed him up again and sent him home to die. A few weeks later his sister brought him a publication containing an account of the Hoxsey treatment. His brother, who accompanied him to the clinic, tells you: "What do we have to lose?

Even if this treatment doesn't cure him, at least he has a chance to fight for his life."

No. 3—The middle-aged woman from Ohio says she contracted cancer 12 years ago and submitted to amputation of the right breast, followed by 16 x-ray treatments. Last year nodules suddenly appeared in the scar of the operation. A biopsy revealed the recurrence of cancer. She received 18 more x-ray treatments, was burned so severely that the skin flaked off her chest and back. Four months later the nodules reappeared. She tells you she has severe pains in her right arm, shows you the swollen glands of her neck. The doctors have told her she is incurable, suggested intensive x-ray to build a wall of dead tissue around the cancer and confine it. She has refused, declaring she would rather die than go through more agony. A neighbor who once took the Hoxsey treatment recommended our clinic.

No. 4—This young fellow works for an oil company in Houston. He shows you a black spot about the size of a silver dollar on his upper right arm. The company doctor said it was an unmistakable *melanocarcinoma* ("black cancer," the most deadly type of the disease) and declared the entire arm would have to be amputated. Even then his chance of recovery is slim, since this type of cancer spreads rapidly and other areas of his body probably already are invaded. A semi-professional ball player, the patient says if he had to die he'd rather be buried "all in one piece." The sports columns of a local paper carried his story. The day after it appeared he received a phone call from a former Hoxsey patient, urging him to come to this clinic for treatment.

The above are actual first-person accounts from case histories taken in one day by the nurse who interviews patients at our clinic. They represent a fair cross-section of those who come to us for treatment.

Cancer victims come to us because they're unwilling to accept as final a death sentence handed them by their own doctors.

Or because they refuse to submit to mutilation by knife or searing irradiation without any certainty that this will save their lives.

Or because they already have tried conventional methods, and these have failed.

They come to the clinic as a last resort, like drowning men clutching at a straw, because they don't want to die.

We don't pretend to cure all of them. The vast majority are advanced and even terminal cases by the time we get them. Many come to us after the disease already has spread through the body; after surgery or irradiation has so impaired circulation of the blood to the affected areas that our treatment cannot reach them; after ravages of the disease, or previous treatment, have so damaged vital organs and functions that even if the cancer were eradicated the patient still would die. No cure, however effective, can regenerate vital tissue once it has been destroyed.

Nevertheless we believe we cure a far greater percentage of cases treated than is cured by any other method at present known to science.

That is a tall claim. In subsequent chapters I propose to document it thoroughly enough to convince any fair and impartial reader, layman or professional.

CHAPTER TWO

Portrait of the Killer

As a cause of death cancer is unique in that it attacks all forms of life: vegetable, animal and human. And it strikes down human beings of all races, types, ages, geographic locations and economic status. Long considered primarily an affliction of middle and old age, it now occupies second place in frequency as the major cause of death in infants from birth to five years of age, and is the chief cause of death (from disease) in children between the ages of five and 19. Some 17 percent of all cancer of the breast occurs among women under 40.

From the cradle to the grave every man, woman and child on earth is stalked by this killer.

Cancer is not a new disease. It was known in Egypt 4500 years ago, in India at least 4000 years ago. An excellent description of it was recorded by Hippocrates nearly 2400 years ago; he called the hard, rapidly-growing swellings *karkinos,* or *karkinoma* (from which the modern term *carcinoma* derives). More than 1700 years ago another famous physician of antiquity, Galen, observed: *"Just as a crab's feet extend from every part of its body, so in this disease the veins* (he meant lymph glands) *are distended, forming a similar figure."* He gave the crab-like disease the name it now bears, *cancer.*

Over the centuries we've learned a lot about this disease, and its development. Yet today if you ask the average layman what cancer is, he will tell you only that it's a "malignant growth." He has no more idea of the nature, characteristics, origin or development of that growth than he has of the craters in the moon. Cancer victims themselves are singularly uninformed on the subject. I am constantly amazed to discover how little the vast majority of our patients know about the loathsome enemy that is consuming their flesh and vital organs.

In order to demonstrate why surgery, x-ray and radium offer little hope to cancer sufferers, and to explain the scientific basis for the Hoxsey method, it may be well to start with a brief review of the biological process that characterizes the development of this highly malignant disease.

Growth is one of the fundamental activities of life. All living matter begins its existence as a single living cell which reproduces itself by division. As the reproductive process continues, tissue and organs are formed. The number of cells increase with remarkable speed between conception and birth. Although still quite rapid after birth, the rate of increase gradually slows down as the organism approaches maturity. After maturity, cellular production normally continues only at a rate sufficient to repair or replace damaged, worn-out or destroyed cells.

Thus normal growth is orderly, controlled and predictable. And normalcy (or health) in the adult body depends to a very large extent' on maintaining a balance between cellular supply and demand.

Sometimes one or more new-born cells suddenly manifest a strange immunity to the chemical forces that regulate growth. Endowed with extraordinary energy, they divide at a speed that may equal or even exceed that normally occurring before birth. In total disregard of the natural laws of structure and function they run riot, invade surrounding cells, create tissue which serves no useful purpose and for which there is no room in the organism.

Such centers of outlaw growth are known as *tumors*. They are autonomous new growths (*neoplasms*) which show different degrees of disorganization and lack of control.

Some, such as warts, wens and moles, are content to remain in their immediate locale. They may become quite large and cause considerable distress, but they never break loose and invade other areas of the body. They are known medically as *benign tumors*.

Others are more vicious. Not satisfied with merely invading their immediate neighbors, they break loose, infiltrate the blood stream or lymph system, are carried to distant parts of the body. There they set up new lawless colonies and continue their ruthless propagation. Eventually they reach vital organs, disrupt the body's intricate and delicate balance, interrupt normal functions. The brakes on growth provided by nature have failed, the human machine careens downgrade to destruction. These groups of gangster cells are known as *malignant tumors*.

The superficial resemblance between benign and malignant tumors (especially in the early stages of the latter) is so close that it is practically impossible to tell one from another, except under the microscope. Patients often come to the Hoxsey clinic half scared to death because two or three doctors have clinically diagnosed a swelling as cancerous, yet on examination we find that it is non-malignant. The average general practitioner sees perhaps 100 cases of cancer in a lifetime; our doctors see 500 to 600 every week.

Under the microscope the cells of a benign tumor look exactly like the ordinary, adult cells of the tissue or organ in which they arise. Cancer cells, however, are unlike any normal adult cell in the body. In appearance they are young and undifferentiated, strikingly similar to the cells encountered in the embryo shortly after conception; they have not become specialized, or adapted to any particular function. A malignant tumor of a gland, for example, does not develop a duct for the discharge of secretions. It does not develop a nerve connection, and is not under the control of the general nervous system.

Cancer may be described as cellular anarchy. Its outstanding characteristics are purposeless, never-ending, unrestrained and uncontrollable cell production, and the ability of these lawless cells to migrate (*metastasize*) to other sites in the body and so extend their destructive activities.

It is important to note that the disease always arises in a local site within a normal organ or tissue. And that it begins as a specific malignant cell which multiplies by dividing itself, not by converting neighboring cells into cancer cells. It may originate in any part of the human body, and each particular section of the body produces a specific type of cancer which retains its original character, wherever it may migrate. For example, lung metastasis of a breast cancer will consist of breast cells, not lung cells.

More than 300 different types of human cancer have been discovered. Generally they are classified in one of two categories:

Carcinoma, the most common, originates in the epithelial tissues. Typical sites are the skin, breast, uterus, stomach, rectum, intestines and ovaries. It metastasizes almost entirely in the lymph channels, varies extremely in virulence.

Sarcoma originates in the structural framework. Typical sites are the bones, muscle, tendons, testicles, kidney. It metastasizes almost entirely through the blood vessels, and its rate of growth usually is more rapid than the other.

But there are as many subdivisions as there are organs and tissues in the body, the particular origin of each indicated by a prefix (*adenocarcinoma, fibrosarcoma,* etc.) *Leukemia* is a malignancy of the cell groups whose function is to produce white blood cells; cancer of the cells that produce the pigmentation of the skin is called *malignant melanoma.*

Each type of cancer has its own pattern of growth, development and virulence; no two tumors behave in exactly the same manner. A fibroid of the uterus may grow for 40 years without attracting attention and without metastasis; acute leukemia may prove fatal within a month. Basal cell tumors of the skin are relatively benign, seldom metastasize and yield readily to treatment; malignant melanomas metastasize at a very early stage, frequently before they are noticed, and the survival rate is very low.

Indeed the appearance and behavior of these "wild" cells, even within a single type, are so varied that many medical authorities hold cancer is not a single disease, but a large family of diseases having in common the attribute of uncontrolled cell division.

What is the basic cause of cancer?

Galen, about 200 A.D., thought that it was due to stagnation of the "black bile" which, he said, was one of the "four humors" of the body. Paracelsus in the 17th century maintained that it was caused by a concentration of mineral salts. Physicians of the early 18th century believed it resulted from coagulation and degeneration of the lymph. In 1775 Dr. Pott observed that English chimney sweeps developed cancer of the scrotum as the result of constant contact with tar-soaked trousers, and speculated that this disease might be caused by some irritant in the tar. Many of his colleagues thought that cancer generally resulted from a severe blow, others that it was hereditary.

Doctors were fumbling in the dark. Little more than a hundred years ago, chemists and pathologists settled down to work with flasks, test tubes and microscopes in laboratories in various parts of the world, and the age of scientific research began.

We know that cancer is not contagious. There is no record in medical history of anyone contracting this disease because of intimate contact with a victim.

Can it be inherited?

In 1907 it was shown that the offspring of mice with cancer of the breast or lung are more likely to develop the same malignancy than the offspring of non-cancerous animals. Exhaustive experiments with rodents over the ensuing years have shown that this is also true of cancer of the uterus, connective tissue, liver and white blood cells. By carefully selecting and breeding together cancerous stock, in about 5 generations certain strains of mice were produced in which 100 percent of each litter ultimately developed malignancy of the same organ. One strain exclusively reproduced breast cancer, another intestinal cancer, etc.

Such experiments led to a widespread belief in medical circles that heredity plays a determining role in the origin and development of human cancer. Actually they proved nothing of the sort. Our society deliberately discourages human inbreeding, and a cancerous (or noncancerous) ancestry in common is not a prerequisite to human mating.

Statistics on the incidence of human cancer are uncertain and confusing. Recent studies show that cancer of the breast is three times more prevalent among the daughters of women with this type of disease than among the general population. However others even more recent indicate that cancer patients have no higher percentage of cancerous relatives than do non-cancerous patients.

A survey of cases at the Hoxsey Clinic indicates that less than half of our patients have a history of cancer in the immediate family.

As of now, the most that can be said authoritatively on this subject is that a predisposition to a particular type of cancer *may* be inherited.

Today three theories as to the cause of cancer have gained considerable support and are under intensive investigation:

1—Chronic irritation,
2—Virus infection,
3—Hormone disturbances.

Widespread scientific interest in the chronic irritation theory, first proposed by Pott in 1775, was revived in 1915 when two Japanese pathologists succeeded in inducing skin cancer in rabbits by painting the animals' ears with coal tar. The active cancer-producing irritant (*carcinogen*) in tar was isolated 17 years later by British chemists. It is a compound known as *benzpyrene*.

Since then more than 20 organic and inorganic irritants capable of producing malignancy in human tissue have been found.

Dentists, orthopedic surgeons, radium and x-ray technicians regularly exposed to radiation are particularly susceptible to skin cancer. Workers in the dye industry often develop cancer of the bladder as the result of constant exposure to aniline and other chemicals. Cancer of the respiratory tract is common among workers exposed to fumes and vapors of chromium, nickel, arsenic and mineral pigments. Workers exposed to benzol may develop leukemia, those exposed to coal tar and arsenic compounds often contract multiple cancers of the skin. Cancer of the tongue or cheek often is attributed to ill-fitting dental plates, cancer of the lip to the constant pressure of a hot pipe-stem, cancer of the oesophagus to the habit of swallowing hot liquids. Seamen, farmers and others constantly exposed to the hot rays of the sun often get skin cancer.

Could chronic irritation be responsible for the alarming increase of cancer of the lung during the past 20 years?

Some researchers, noting that lung cancer is more prevalent in industrial areas than in rural districts, came to the conclusion that pollution of the air by industry and transportation is responsible. They held that the smoke of furnaces and factories, the exhaust of gasoline and diesel engines, dust from rubber tires and asphalted and oiled roads waft a heavy concentration of carcinogens into the air and thence into the lungs of the population.

But when laboratory animals were exposed to the same carcinogens in even more concentrated form, a raft of conflicting data resulted. Principally because it is almost impossible to find animals which develop lung tumors comparable to those in man.

Other investigators, observing that the consumption of cigarettes in this country has increased fourfold during the past 20 years (in 1953 an average of 187 packs of cigarettes were sold for every American over the age of 15) undertook more than a dozen independent studies to determine whether there was any connection between excessive smoking and lung cancer.

Last year (1954) the American Cancer Society made public the spectacular results of one such study, a 20-months project covering nearly 5,000 men aged 50 to 70, their smoking habits and the cause of their death. It showed that people who smoke a pack or more of cigarettes per day are 10 times more likely to develop lung cancer than those who never smoke. And those who smoke less than a pack a day are 4½ times more likely to develop the disease than those who abstain entirely.

A second report this year covering the deaths of more than 8,000 men, resulted in the following conclusions:

1—Lung cancer is rare among men who have never smoked;
2—The death rate from lung cancer increases with the number of cigarettes consumed by the individual, but

the increase is appreciable even among those who smoke fewer than 10 cigarettes daily;

3—Among those who smoke two packs or more daily, lung cancer accounts for one in 8 deaths. In the general population it accounts for only one in 30 deaths;

4—Regardless of whether they live in city or rural areas, the rate is high among smokers and low among non-smokers.

This report aroused considerable alarm among smokers, and consternation in the tobacco industry. Several prominent medical authorities immediately registered their sharp dissent. One of these, Dr. W. C. Heuper of the National Cancer Institute, contends:

"The cigarette theory is almost entirely based on statistical data having at best circumstantial value and being in part of questionable origin."

Does the good doctor suggest that the American Cancer Society is a "questionable" source? Heaven forbid! And the controversy rages on.

(Incidentally a survey of case histories at the Hoxsey Clinic indicates that smoking plays little or no part in the incidence of lung cancer among our patients. This is especially true of women who have come to us with this type of malignancy.)

One conspicuous discrepancy of the chronic irritation theory is the fact that many extremely heavy smokers never get cancer of the lung; many workers exposed constantly to various carcinogens never get cancer of the bladder, respiratory tract etc.; many pipe addicts never get cancer of the lip. On the other hand there are numerous cancer victims whose history reveals no evidence of chronic irritation.

The virus infection theory first aroused intense interest in 1911 when Rous succeeded in transmitting sarcoma from one fowl to another of the same species by inoculating the latter with a cell-free extract of the original tumor. Other researchers successfully completed similar experiments on frogs, domestic rabbits, rats and mice. It seemed obvious that a virus must carry the infection from one animal to another.

Some 25 years later Bittner apparently confirmed this. He demonstrated that new-born mice, suckled by mothers with cancer of the breast, at maturity themselves developed cancer of the breast. Heredity played no part in this phenomenon. For when the same mothers were given foster-children of a cancer-free strain to suckle, the latter also came down with cancer of the breast.

Recently, scientists with the aid of the newly-developed electronic microscope actually were able to see small spherical particles in samples of milk obtained from mice with cancer of the breast. Similar micro-organisms were observed in tumor extracts and cell cultures from mice with cancer of the breast, and when purified preparations of these were injected into susceptible mice, cancer of the breast occurred. Identical particles have been observed in human milk, and it is noted that their presence coincides roughly with a history of cancer in the donor's family.

However, while cancer can be transmitted from animal to animal within the same species, it cannot be transmitted from one species to another—from a mouse to a rat, for example. Attempts to transmit it from one human to another by means of an extract of cancer cells or a solution of milk particles have failed. And efforts to isolate an infectious virus in human cancer likewise have failed.

In short, if cancer is due to a virus infection, it is entirely different from any other infection known to medicine. Therefore most authorities in the field refuse to accept this theory.

For many years endocrinologists have noted a striking similarity in chemical structure between hormones produced by the human body and chemically-produced carcinogens. The cancer-producing agent in tar, for example, is also a component of such glandular substances as cholesterol. Methyl cholanthrene, one of the most powerful of all carcinogens used in animal experiments, is a constituent of bile. Testosterone, which also incites cancer, is a synthetic duplicate of a secretion of the male sex glands.

Dr. L. F. Fieser of Harvard University, who has done considerable research on such substances, has become convinced that abnormal metabolism (chemical changes incidental to life and growth in the cells) may stimulate certain glands to abnormal activity and transform their secretions into cancer-producing substances.

This theory is not necessarily in conflict with either the chronic irritation or the virus infection theories; in fact it complements them and offers a logical explanation of their basic effect upon the human organism. As Dr. G. S. Sperti put it, more than 10 years ago:

". . . cancer-causing agents have the power to injure large numbers of cells and to keep them injured over a long period of time, resulting in the secretion of a large and continuous quantity of growth factor and an unbalance in metabolism. This may be the cause of cancer."

As we shall see in succeeding chapters, the imbalance in body chemistry and cell metabolism is one of the key factors in the development of cancer—and the primary target of the Hoxsey treatment.

CHAPTER THREE

Why Surgery, X-ray and Radium Fail

Wₕₑₙ we examine current methods of treating cancer, we venture into an area of bitter controversy and acrimonious debate where most medical angels fear to tread.

An article in the *Saturday Evening Post* (Dec. 21, 1946) states that *"a doctor who claims to know an effective treatment for cancer not involving surgery, radium or x-ray is an ipso facto quack."*

As recently as July 1952 a Federal Circuit Court in Texas handed down an amazing decision (we will discuss it at length later) which declares flatly: *"Qualified experts recognize that the only treatment for internal cancer is surgery, x-ray, radium and radioactive products."*

That today is the arbitrary position of organized medicine. Those who stray off the beaten path of approved knowledge no longer are burned at the stake as they were in the Middle Ages. Nevertheless highly reputable doctors who experiment with, advocate or use treatments for cancer other than those approved by the AMA are violently denounced as quacks, expelled from their professional organizations, banned from hospitals and fired from their jobs, often without any real investigation of the merits of the treatment in question.

For example: Dr. Andrew C. Ivy, once vice-president of the University of Illinois and head of its medical school, the largest in the nation; former Executive Director of the National Advisory Cancer Council; director of the American Cancer Society. When he began to experiment with the drug *Krebiozen* on cancer patients he was suspended from the Chicago Medical Society, denounced as naive and misguided, forced to resign his various official and professional positions.

For example: Dr. Robert E. Lincoln, suspended from the AMA and hounded to death because he persisted in using a bacteriophage in the treatment of cancer.

For example: Dr. William F. Koch, M.D. and Ph.D., former instructor in histology and embryology at the University of Michigan and professor of physiology at the Detroit Medical College. When he developed a drug called *"Glyoxylide"* and used it in the treatment of cancer he was persecuted as a quack, prosecuted by the Government and eventually forced into voluntary exile in Brazil.

The list of doctors who suffered a similar fate because they pioneered unauthorized cancer research or treatment is too long for further particularization.

Exactly how effective are surgery, radium and x-ray in the treatment of cancer?

In 1953 no less an authority than Dr. Cornelius P. Rhoads, director of the Sloan-Kettering Institute for Cancer Research (a unit of the Memorial Center for Cancer and Allied Diseases, in New York City) admitted publicly that these treatments are *possible* in only 25 percent of all cancer cases! He didn't say how many of the patients treated by these methods recovered. But even the most optimistic figure stated by authorities in the field seldom exceeds 25 percent.

Over the years there has been a tremendous accumulation of weighty and authoritative medical testimony that these treatments are completely ineffectual, except perhaps for skin cancers and other malignancies without metastasis.

A quarter of a century ago Dr. L. Duncan Bulkley, senior surgeon at New York Skin and Cancer Hospital, and an outstanding authority in this disease, stated flatly:

"Cancer is not a surgical disease. Neither surgery, x-ray nor radium has changed in any way whatever the ultimate mortality of cancer in 40 years. It was 90 percent in 1894; now it is 92 percent."

A few years later Dr. W. A. Dewey, formerly professor of medicine at the University of Michigan, wrote:

"In a practice of nearly 45 years I have yet to see a single case of cancer—save a few semi-malignant epitheliomata—cured by surgery, x-ray or radium."

Dr. Ernest A. Codman, a nationally known surgeon and registrar of the American College of Surgeons, was even more specific. At an AMA conference on March 5, 1924, he declared:

"We have now collected from the most efficient surgeons and hospitals in the country notes on some 400 odd cases of supposed bone sarcoma.

"All of these 400 registered cases, with few exceptions, are records of error or failure.

"I have many of the foremost surgeons and pathologists in the country convicted in their own handwriting of gross errors in these cases.

"Legs have been amputated when they should not have been and left on when they should have been amputated!"

Needless to say, Dr. Codman was never asked to address another AMA meeting.

Dr. Stanley Reimann, director of research at Lankenau Hospital (leading cancer institution of Philadelphia), conducted an extensive survey of cancer cases over a period of years. In a report to a U.S. Senate Committee in 1946 he concluded that those who received no treatment at all lived much longer than those who received surgery, radium or x-ray! And that these treatments actually cause more harm than good to the average victim!

Except for cautery, surgery is the most ancient of all cancer treatments. Leonides, the greatest of all cancer experts of ancient times, used the knife to excise tumors as far back as 180 B.C. The methods he employed remained in use for nearly 2,000 years. In 1839 Dr. John Lizars, professor of the Royal College of Surgeons, developed the doctrine that wherever possible all the lymph tissue in the area of the cancerous growth should also be removed, as a prophylactic against metastasis. This is common practice today in many types of cancer.

Organized medicine considers surgery "the most reliable weapon in the war on cancer." Yet even our brief study of the biological development of the disease should make it obvious that this method can be effective only in the early stages, before the "wild" cells have run riot through the system. For once they spread to distant parts of the body it is impossible to ferret out and remove all of them.

Unfortunately cancer is probably the most difficult of all diseases to diagnose. In its early stages it presents none of the usual dramatic "warning signals," such as pain, discomfort or fever. By the time the first suspicious signs appear the disease frequently is well distributed and entrenched in the victim, vital organs have been seriously damaged, it is too late for surgery.

Moreover cancer is not just an autonomous growth, springing from nowhere; it is the result of some mysterious abnormal condition in the body. Cut out the growth and the abnormal condition that produced it will persist and often produce another outbreak.

As the eminent Dr. Robert Bell observed in an article entitled "Cancer is a Blood Disease and Must Be Treated as Such" (*N.Y. Medical Record,* March 18, 1922):

> "Cancer is rooted in every drop of blood in the body and we may as well expect to stop the growing of apples by picking them off trees, or to stop the springing of dandelions by cutting off the blossoms and leaving the root in the ground, as to expect to destroy malignancy in the human body by attacking the outward growth."

Dr. Bell then was head of the Cancer Research Department of Battersea Hospital (England) as well as vice-president of the International Society for Cancer Research. Despite these exalted positions his unorthodox view that cancer is a blood disease, and especially his attacks upon surgery and irradiation as ineffective in the treatment of cancer, led officials of the British Medical Society to stigmatize him publicly as a "quack." He promptly sued for libel and slander, won a court decision and damages totaling £10,000 (nearly $50,000 at that time).

Numerous other medical authorities agree that the treatment of cancer by surgery and/or irradiation usually is followed by another outcrop of the disease.

Thirty years ago Dr. G. Everett Field, director of the Radium Institute of New York, observed:

"Blindly we have been attacking cancer in its advanced stages for many generations with surgical effort, only to find prompt recurrence after removal."

Dr. Alexander Braunschwig, attending surgeon at Memorial Hospital in New York, recently told the International College of Surgeons that *about 40 percent of the pelvic cancer victims* (who survive the radical operation) *die within a year because of a recurrence of the cancer.* The good doctor's figures are extremely conservative, by comparison with other statistics.

In the standard medical text, *Tumors of the Breast,* Dr. Max Cutler and Sir G. Lenthal Cheatle assert:

"Of the cases entering the hospital with recurrence after operation, only 3 percent are alive and well. The addition of preoperative or postoperative prophylactic x-ray treatment to radical surgery gave no greater percentage of five-year successful results."

Significantly, few cancer specialists speak of a "cure" in connection with surgery. If the patient survives five years after the operation with no further indication of cancer, he is considered "clinically cured." Doctors talk of *"five year cures," "ten year cures"* etc., because they know the disease may flare up again at any time. At the Hoxsey Clinic we have treated cases in which cancer nodules suddenly reappeared in the scars of a radical operation performed as many as twelve years previously for the same disease.

In the past few years a sharp trend toward more radical operations has been noted, especially in cases of cancer of the pelvic organs (uterus, bladder, prostate) and cancer of the stomach and breast. One of the few distinguished medical men with courage enough to denounce this vicious practice is Dr. O. Theron Clagett, famous Mayo Clinic surgeon. On March 1st of this year (1955) he told the Society of Graduate Surgeons of Los Angeles County:

> "We are in a terrible trend toward too fast and radical surgery. More conservatism and fewer quickly decided upon radical operations are in order for the future. You may find that a cancer operation that will save a few weeks or months of a man's life may cost so much that his children can't go to college. You have to be sure that the most radical operation will make a man live more and not less comfortably."

He asserted bluntly that radical surgery is not the answer to cancer (except possibly in breast cases) because the knife *"fails to remove all possible routes of spreading."* And later, in an interview with the press, he voiced an opinion which only a few years ago would have been regarded by his colleagues as rank heresy, and almost certainly would have gotten him suspended from the AMA.

He stated openly that he was certain cancer eventually would be cured by drugs! He declared:

> "If I were a young man I wouldn't go in for surgery. The best thing now would be to get a college degree in chemistry before getting a medical degree. Future health lies more in the laps of the internal medical men than in the hands of us surgeons."

Such frankness unfortunately is all too rare in authoritative medical circles. Physicians continue to recommend the knife to cancer patients even when the diagnosis is not absolutely certain, and the chances of survival (in the event the diagnosis proves correct) are very slim.

In a speech in New Orleans two years ago Dr. Alton Ochsner, former president of the American College of Surgeons and of the American Cancer Society, stated: *"Any possibility of stomach cancer should be treated as though it really were cancer. Most of the stomach should be taken out."*

In practically the same breath he admitted that *"only from 5 to 10 percent"* of cases of stomach cancer are saved by this radical operation!

(Incidentally, Dr. Ochsner is chairman of the department of surgery at the Tulane University School of Medicine, and as such shapes the future thinking of a rising generation of doctors.)

Why do surgeons continue to perform such operations, when they know they are futile?

An illuminating comment on the subject by no less an authority than Dr. Paul R. Hawley, director of the American College of Surgeons, appeared in *U.S. News and World Report* (Feb. 20, 1953). The reporter quoted him as stating that people *"would be shocked, I think, at the amount of unnecessary surgery that is performed."* Asked why a doctor should perform such an operation, he replied succinctly: *"Money!"*

Asked if he really thought doctors went to such lengths for filthy lucre, Dr. Hawley snapped: *"I don't just think it, I know it. And I can prove it!"*

As for x-ray and radium, it is customary to hail these as "modern developments" (x-ray was first applied to cancer of the skin in 1896, radium in 1903). Actually both are merely refinements of barbaric treatments of antiquity. About 4,000 years ago the Chinese used *moxa,* a smoldering fire, to destroy tumors; Hippocrates used a white-hot iron. In x-ray and radium doctors found a new kind of fire with which to combat cancer. Moreover rays penetrate to inner reaches of the body usually not accessible to ordinary methods of cautery.

The cauterizing effect of rays emanating from a vacuum tube through which an electric current is passed was discovered accidentally. Severe burns suffered by early workers with x-ray gave Dr. Emil Grubbe the idea that this destructive energy might be beneficially employed to destroy malignant growths. It is ironic to note that Dr. Grubbe's new method of cancer therapy encountered bitter opposition from leading doctors of his generation—the predecessors of the same medical hierarchy which now embraces x-ray therapy and just as bitterly fights advanced methods like the Hoxsey treatment. It took 37 years for x-ray treatment to win the approval of the American College of Surgeons.

The discovery of radium therapy was equally accidental. Dr. Becqueral, the great French physicist and radiation pioneer, took a tube of the newly-discovered crystals to a lecture to London. For safe-keeping, he carried it in his vest pocket. On his return to Paris he found on his abdomen a red spot which gradually increased in size over the weeks, with considerable destruction of tissue.

This gave other experimenters a clue. They enclosed radium in a shielded screen and focussed the so-called "gamma" rays on skin cancer. It destroyed them, all right. About 1920 the first "radium bombs" were used against internal cancer. Long, thin, hollow needles were thrust into cancerous masses in the breast, womb and

other parts of the body, and through these tubes tiny
radium pellets were shot into the malignancy. This technique still is employed on various types of internal cancer.

Both x-rays and radium kill cells by bringing about a
minor atomic explosion—they produce intense ioniza-
tion within the cells, knocking the electrons out of the
atoms.

Do x-ray and radium cure cancer?

The most ardent exponents of these treatments acknowledge that their therapeutic effect is extremely limited. For example Dr. Edward Podolsky, a faculty member of the New York Medical College, writes:

> "Often it is impossible to give a large enough dose of
> x-rays to kill the cancer without harming the patient. The
> best that can be done at present with x-rays is to cure or
> benefit about 15 percent of the patients treated—about one
> out of six."

As Dr. Francis Carter Wood, professor emeritus at St.
Luke's Hospital (New York City) and vice-president of
the organization that later became the American Cancer
Society, observed:

> "Radium will not cure cancer. It only destroys cancer
> tissues within a certain radius, but it does not drive the
> disease from the blood."

Dr. William S. Bainbridge, former surgical director of
New York City's Children's Hospital and of Manhattan
State Hospital, in 1946 told a U.S. Senate Committee:

> "While there are some who still believe in the efficiency
> of radiation as a cure, my skepticism with regard to its value

is being increasingly sustained. Even with the best technic of today, its curative effect on a real cancer is questionable."

In 1953 Dr. Ross Golden, professor of radiology at Columbia University College of Physicians and Surgeons, presented a paper at a four-day session of the Dallas Southern Clinical Society in which he declared that radiation is no more the answer to cancer than is surgery. He added:

"What somebody needs to do is find out why cancer develops and eliminate the cause. Radiation does not treat the cause."

One serious objection to irradiation is indicated in an editorial in the Michigan *Annals of Internal Medicine* (May 1930):

"As to the curative results from x-ray and radium irradiation, these methods of treatment of malignant neoplasms have proved very disappointing. Particularly is the irradiation of the affected area after operative removal of the neoplasm now being advised against, as some workers believe that such irradiation favors the occurrence of metastases."

The inexpert application of irradiation, far from curing this disease, frequently causes considerable damage to normal tissue. It affects not only the tumor itself but also the vessels that feed it, obliterating them and producing early necrosis. It causes serious burns and ulcers, resulting in the malformation and malfunction of normal tissue.

A graphic description of what may happen was written 30 years ago by Dr. E. C. Folkmar, editor of *Scientific Therapy and Practical Research:*

"It is no wonder that when a physician has attended a patient with an extensive necrosis following the application of radium needles, or has seen the entire side of a face below the eye, even extending down into the neck and part of the jaw, slough away some months after the injection of radium 'seeds' into these tissues, that he should say: 'Never again will I recommend the use of radium. The remedy seems to be worse than the disease.'"

In 1938, when the British Ministry of Health placed orders for nearly $1 million worth of radium for the treatment of cancer, the authoritative English publication the *Medical World* (Dec. 2, 1938) commented:

"This radium is by far the least important of the available treatments for cancer. It is an extremely dangerous agent causing great pain and often severe injuries to those who are treated with it . . . it is in no sense a desirable treatment for the great majority of cases of cancer."

Seven years later (July 7, 1945) this publication was still of the same opinion. It declared:

"The average practitioner is no friend to deep x-ray therapy for malignant disease, because he has usually seen more than one case in which death has been rendered more horrible than it would have been if the disease had taken its normal course. Nor is he convinced that radium is curative in any but a very restricted series of cases."

In 1946 Dr. Herman J. Muller, world-renowned scientist and Nobel Prize winner, warned a Senate Committee: *"There is no dosage of x-ray so low as to be without risk of producing harmful mutation."*

Indeed it has been established that both x-ray and radium themselves actually produce cancer.

The official publication of the British Medical Society, the *Lancet* (Nov. 12, 1938) stated that rectal ulcers often resulted from treatment (with radium) or cancer of the cervix, and that cancer of the uterus was a possible result of treatment (by radium) of post-menopausal bleeding.

And in 1946 *Cancer*, official publication of the American Cancer Society, published a 20-page report by five prominent medical researchers stating that both x-ray and gamma rays may cause sarcoma of the bone.

All of which led Sir Leonard Hill, the great British physiologist, to write in 1939:

"The world would, I think, be little the worse off if all the radium in the country now buried in deep holes for security in bombings were to remain there."

Thus there is conclusive evidence that x-ray and radium have no place in the treatment of cancer. At best they are palliative rather than curative; they represent another attempt to deal with the symptoms rather than the disease itself. They weaken the body, sap its resistance, if improperly administered may hasten death.

As a matter of fact many cancer patients die because of too extensive therapy, either radiological or surgical. Their deaths can be directly attributed to functional or anatomical deformities produced by these treatments.

According to organized medicine the approved treatments—surgery and irradiation—will cure most cases of cancer if the disease is diagnosed soon enough. The need for early detection of the disease is constantly emphasized, we are constantly exhorted to get a complete physical check up at least once a year (and if over 35, at least every six months).

No one can quarrel with the statement that early detection of a deadly disease vastly improves the chances of a cure. But the fact remains that this is a subtle and stealthy enemy, and that present-day methods of cancer diagnosis are not nearly as effective as medical propaganda would have us believe.

For example, our Congressmen and Senators get regular physical check ups and are under almost constant medical observation. Yet within four years no fewer than five Senators—Arthur Vandenburg, of Michigan, Robert Taft of Ohio, Brien McMahon of Connecticut, and Lester Hunt of Wyoming—all died of cancer. In each case the most thorough physical examination at regular intervals failed to detect any trace of the deadly disease until it was far advanced. And in each case surgery and irradiation by the best specialists in the nation failed to save the victim's life.

Early detection is obviously impossible at present in many if not most cases of cancer. Even if it were possible it would not be the answer to the problem. The only hope to cope with this terrible disease is to seek a truly effective cure and preventative.

Now both surgery and irradiation are based on the theory that tumors are autonomous growths on an otherwise healthy organism, something like parasitic growths on trees. Cut away the malignancy or burn it off, and the organism will flourish again.

Nearly half a century ago a handful of earnest scientists, convinced by vital statistics that these treatments were not effective, began to suspect that tumors are not entirely autonomous growths but rather symptoms of a sick organism. They set to work in their laboratories and came up with a number of important discoveries.

In the 1920s Dr. Otto Warburg, a Nobel Prize winner, demonstrated that the metabolism (chemical changes incidental to life and growth) of cancerous tissue differs radically from that of normal tissue. The latter acquires its nourishment from oxidation, and usually dies if deprived of oxygen. But cancerous tissue subsists by a process in which cell-nutritive substances are broken down by specialized chemicals, much as food is broken down in ordinary digestion, and so needs little or no oxygen to exist. Subsequent experiments established that normal animal tissue may become cancerous if deprived of oxygen at long intervals.

Since the blood provides cells of the body with oxygen, Warburg's discovery indicated that the condition of the blood stream must play an important part in the development of cancer. This is substantiated by the fact that malignant tumors frequently are found in or near scars, at the side of ulcers, in atrophied organs and in other places where the blood supply is poor.

Other researchers noted an increase of alkalinity in the blood plasma of most cancer patients. Experimenting with marine cells, they discovered that when the alkaline content of sea water is increased even slightly, cell division is accelerated; on the other hand when acid is introduced into the water, cell division is greatly retarded, or even halted entirely. As frentic cell division is a fundamental characteristic of cancer, they deduced that increased alkalinity in the body may be an important factor in the development of the disease.

Recently it was discovered that the chemistry of the cancer cell nucleus differs considerably in synthesis of amino-acid from that of normal cells.

And only last year a researcher at Southwestern Medical School announced that he had found a factor which regulates the speed with which energy derived from food is transported to the body cells, hence controls the speed of cellular growth. This agent, normally produced by the healthy organism, he called the "Q factor." It allegedly slows down the transfer of energy to the cells. His theory is that cancer patients either have less of this factor in their blood stream than normal, or else have developed a counter-agent which destroys the "Q factor" and thus permits an excessive transfer of energy to the cells.

From these physical and chemical changes, and others too technical to discuss here, one general conclusion can be drawn: basic disturbances in blood chemistry and cell metabolism accompany the development of cancer, if indeed they do not cause it.

This concept received wide publicity at the Sixth International Cancer Congress at São Paulo, Brazil, in 1954. In a paper read before distinguished delegates from all over the world, Dr. Nikolai Blokhin, of the Soviet Academy of Science, declared that Soviet scientists consider cancer due to a number of agents, including chemical and physical factors which *"may bring about alterations in the metabolism and in certain conditions provoke cancer."* Noting that a long series of experiments have shown *"the dependence of the growth of tumors on the general health of the organism,"* he asserted that cancer specialists in his country *"deny that there is complete autonomy*

*of tumor growths and regard cancer as an illness of the
organism as a whole."*

Within the past 5 or 6 years this view has gained wide
acceptance in research laboratories (if not among practicing physicians) throughout the civilized world. As a
result perhaps 85 percent of all cancer research today in
this country is devoted to one aspect or another of a treatment basic to the chemistry of the human body, to chemical substances that are taken internally or are injected
into the body of cancer victims in order to normalize or
halt the abnormal processes taking place there. Most
researchers are convinced that chemotherapy offers the
only real hope for a solution of the great plague.

In 1948 Dr. Cornelius Rhoads of the Sloan Kettering
Institute published a paper in which he conceded a belief
that *"the problem of cancer is insoluble by any existing
technic."* Then he went on to voice an opinion which he
himself called "radical" and *"contrary to general scientific opinion."* He wrote:

"Though it is true, and must be completely understood,
that the chemical restraint of cancer at the moment is rare,
most incomplete and wholly transient, *it does exist.* This fact,
coupled with experimental evidence, brings us an all-im-
portant conclusion. Cancer is not necessarily a wholly uncontrollable growth which must destroy or be destroyed.
Real hope exists that other and less mutilating measures for
control can be found."

In the ensuing years this opinion has become not so
radical. Only last year Dr. Charles S. Cameron, Executive
Director of the American Cancer Society, guardedly
broadcast over the radio the significant statement that

"when a cure for cancer is discovered," in all probability
it will be chemical!

Yet as late as last April (1955) no less an informed
authority than the U.S. Surgeon General, Dr. Leonard
A. Scheele, sent a letter to Congressman Antoni N. Sadlak
in which he stated positively:

> "As you are undoubtedly aware, the only recognized
> methods of treatment which can cure cancer are surgery
> and irradiation by x-ray or radium . . ."

The Surgeon General knows full well that neither surgery nor irradiation can cure cancer after it has metastasized. At the time he wrote this letter he had in his
possession a secret report by the Committee on Chemotherapy of the National Cancer Council (a Government
agency) in cooperation with the American Cancer Society, the National Cancer Institute (another Government agency) and the Damon Runyon Cancer Fund—a
report so secret that on its front cover appears a warning
that *the information contained herein is not for publication or publication reference."*

The report is prefaced by the following statement:

> "This program was inaugurated because of the conviction
> of the Committee that cures for many different kinds of
> cancer will be produced by research in this field (Chemo-
> therapy) . . ."

Why has this report—paid for by Government funds—
never been released to the public?

Publicly these organizations insist that surgery and
irradiation are the only effective cures for cancer. Privately, however, they concede that the only real hope
for an effective cure lies in chemotherapy.

At the same time they persistently refuse to make a fair and impartial scientific test of "unorthodox" methods based on chemotherapy. And they gang up to persecute, prosecute and destroy any individual or institution —like the Hoxsey Clinic—which attempts to treat cancer by chemotherapeutic methods.

The victims of this monstrous hoax are the American people. It already has cost us millions of lives. If it is permitted to continue, it may cost you your life!

CHAPTER FOUR

The Hoxsey Treatment

T<small>HE</small> Hoxsey method essentially is chemotherapy. For more than 50 years my father and I have been treating cancer in human beings—not in mice or rats—with a great degree of success by means of chemical compounds and without the use of surgery, radium or x-ray.

We consider cancer a systemic disease. We don't pretend to know its fundamental cause (no one else does, either, at this writing). But we are convinced that without exception it occurs only in the presence of a profound physiological change in the constituents of body fluids and a consequent chemical imbalance in the organism. This concept, based on extensive practical experience in treating thousands of cancer cases, is in full accord with medically-accepted research outlined in the previous chapter.

For example, a boy bites his tongue in football practice and a sore appears; later it turns out that he has cancer of the tongue. In the course of the same year hundreds of other boys undoubtedly bit their tongues in precisely the same fashion, yet they did not develop cancer. It would appear obvious that in this case the bite was merely the mechanism that triggered the outbreak of the disease. Its real cause must be sought elsewhere, in the basic body chemistry and cell metabolism of the afflicted lad.

We believe that the organism's attempt to adapt itself to the new and abnormal environment produced by the chemical imbalance causes certain changes (mutations) in newly born cells of the body. The mutated cells differ radically in appearance and function from their parent cells. Eventually a viciously competent cell evolves which finds the new environment eminently suitable to survival and rapid self-reproduction. These cells are what is known as cancer.

It follows that if the constitution of body fluids can be normalized and the original chemical balance in the body restored, the environment again will become unfavorable for the survival and reproduction of these cells, they will cease to multiply and eventually they will die. Then if vital organs have not been too seriously damaged by the malignancy (or by surgery or irradiation) the entire organism will recover normal health.

That in brief is the theory of the Hoxsey treatment. We are convinced that cancer cannot be cured successfully as an isolated phenomenon, unrelated to basic body processes. We attempt to get at the roots of the disorder, rather than deal merely with its end result. Our primary effort is to restore the body to physiological normalcy.

We have a basic medicine which, taken orally, accomplishes this purpose. It stimulates the elimination of toxins which are poisoning the system, thereby corrects the abnormal blood chemistry and normalizes cell metabolism. Its ingredients are not secret. It contains potassium iodide combined with some or all of the following inorganic substances, as the individual case may demand: licorice, red clover, burdock root, stillingia root, barberis root, poke root, cascara, Aromatic USP 14, prickly ash bark, buckthorn bark.

It is worth noting that potassium iodide is commonly used in chronic diseases like syphilis to dissolve fibrous tissue in lesions caused by these diseases, and as preparatory action for actual treatment with arsenicals, bismuth and mercury, etc. And that the synthetic anti-coagulant *Dicumarol* derives from spoiled sweet clover.

We prescribe the above medication in all cases of cancer, internal and external. (Except where there is evidence of latent or arrested tuberculosis, in which instance the use of potassium iodide is contraindicated.) The exact ingredients and dosage vary, depending on the individual patient's general condition, the location of the cancer and the extent of previous treatment.

Until recently our medicine was taken in liquid form. Experience demonstrated that it was virtually impossible to standardize dosage in this form; each patient's concept of "a full teaspoon" varied considerably. Therefore last year we arranged with a reputable pharmaceutical firm to put up an improved formula in the form of pills, and these are now standard at our clinic.

In our laboratories we are able to demonstrate that the blood chemistry of patients does undergo definite change as the result of this medicine. And to some extent we also are able to show a change in the activity of the cells, as treatment progresses. Unfortunately the refusal of organzied medicine to permit scientific investigation of our treatment in medically-approved laboratories has prevented any comprehensive study to determine specifically how these changes are brought about. And we have been too busy treating cancer victims—and fighting court battles to keep our clinic open—to spare the time, personnel and facilities for objective study.

In the near future we expect to have a full, scientific report on the Hoxsey treatment and its effects upon blood and cell chemistry in the human body. A non-profit cancer research foundation affiliated with our clinic recently was chartered by the State of Texas. It already has begun work on the above project.

We have another type of medication which we apply locally in external cases. Its purpose is to halt the spread of the disease and speed the *necrosis* (death) of cancer cells. It is employed either as a yellow powder, a red paste or a clear solution, in accordance with the location and type of the cancer. Their formulas are not secret, either. The powder contains arsenic sulphide, yellow precipitate, sulphur and talc; the red paste has antimony trisulphide, zinc chloride and bloodroot; the liquid is Tri-Chloro-Acetic Acid.

All of these are escharotics, and in one form or another were commonly used by the medical profession in the treatment of external cancer long before the development of "more scientific" (and more lucrative) x-ray and radium treatment. We have adopted techniques which result in effective therapy with much less pain and mutilation than that caused by surgery or irradiation. The yellow powder employed in our clinic is highly selective; it reacts only on malignant tissue, does not affect normal tissue. The paste and liquid forms are not selective; however we are able to localize their effects by erecting a vaseline or zinc oxide fence around the area to be treated, thus avoiding damage to normal tissue.

In practice we have found that a small amount of our

compounds, when placed on a large cancerous mass, cause a chain reaction which extends an inch or two beyond the point of application. The mass dies, dries, separates from normal, healthy tissue and falls out.

In fact, organized medicine has conceded that we cure external cancer! (See Chapter 15.)

In addition to the two main groups of medicines I have discussed here, we follow standard medical procedure in the treatment of subsidiary disorders or diseases which may contribute to the normal blood chemistry of patients: for example venereal diseases, kidney ailments, etc.

Thus the Hoxsey method of treating cancer is a combination of three elements: internal medicine, external compounds and supportive treatment.

There is nothing secretive or complicated about it. Any qualified physician who knows the ingredients, has learned the combination and dosage most effective in each type of case and has studied their application in our clinic, can go home and treat his own patients with equal success. A number of doctors, as we shall see later, already have done so.

Now suppose that you are suffering from cancer, and you decide to take the Hoxsey treatment. We do not prescribe medication or send it to patients we have not examined, so you will have to come to the Hoxsey Clinic. What is the procedure, how do our facilities compare with those of orthodox, medically-approved institutions?

You will find the clinic a clean, white, modern building about a mile from the heart of downtown Dallas. It contains 60 rooms including 5 waiting rooms; 10 individual treating rooms; 2 fully-equipped laboratories; a drug dispensary and pharmacy; 3 x-ray units for diagnostic purposes; an emergency room equipped with the latest apparatus for administration of oxygen, plasma and glucose; medical consultation rooms, administration and business offices. Incidentally, our laboratories were approved by the Government for the training of GI veterans.

Our medical staff at this writing consists of 7 physicians headed by Dr. Charles P. Barberee. Under him are Dr. Donald Watt, a certified roentgenologist; Dr. William Stokes, in charge of the external department; Dr. D. C. Logan, Dr. Alfred H. Staffa and Dr. Benjamin H. Harry, all assigned to internal cases. All of these are graduates of leading osteopathic institutions and are duly qualified and licensed to practice medicine without restriction in the State of Texas, as well as other states. Another staff member, Dr. W. F. Pickett, M.D., is a graduate of Baylor University and at this writing still a member of the Dallas County Medical Society. Assisting them are 26 nurses, 8 x-ray technicians and 5 laboratory technicians.

Entering the clinic you sign the register at the reception desk and are directed to the main waiting room, where you will usually find between 100 and 125 patients. Some like you are here for the first time (we process approximately 150 new patients per week); others are in various stages of treatment and report for periodic examination; still others, discharged as cured, have come in for their periodic check-up.

The routine for all new patients begins with an interview by a nurse who takes down your complete medical history. She inquires about previous diagnosis, biopsy and treatment, including the names of doctors and pathologists whom you've consulted. (Nearly all our patients have had a diagnosis of cancer or a biopsy before they arrive, most of them have undergone treatment by surgery, x-ray or radium.) She lists all the symptoms of your complaint such as pain, bleeding, loss of appetite, inablility to sleep, nervousness, etc. She questions you about other illnesses and habits.

When this is completed you are sent to the laboratory for tests. These include blood count and analysis, urinalysis, gastric analysis, bacteriological tests and any others which the doctor who has studied your history considers necessary.

Then you take your turn in one of the x-ray rooms where a full series of x-ray studies is taken. Our x-ray photographic equipment is the finest and most modern available. It includes three Mattern (two 100 x 100 and one 200 x 200) x-ray machines of the latest type, all equipped with fluoroscopes and stereoscopic apparatus. Our darkroom processes an average of 150 films (14 x 17) per day.

Next comes a thorough physical examination by one of our doctors. He will probe the affected areas, attempt to determine by palpation and special examining instruments the location and extent of internal tumors. If yours is an external case, photographs of the lesions are taken from various angles for study and comparison at various stages of treatment.

Your completed record then goes to the doctors' consultation room where it is considered by the clinic's Medical Director, assisted by the examining doctor, the roentgenologist and other members of the staff. Your x-rays go up on a battery of reading boxes, then are carefully studied in the stereoscopic viewer. Our doctors do not accept on faith any previous diagnosis you may have had; their final verdict is based on the sum total of the following:

1. *Your case history.* The symptoms of most cancers are so characteristic that a detailed list of your complaints may be sufficient for a strong presumption of cancer.

2. *Your laboratory tests.* Increased acid phosphates content of the blood is a commonly-accepted indication of cancer of the prostate; excess of albumoses in the blood and urine is a valid sign of myeloma of the bone, etc., etc.

3. *Your x-ray studies.* These are especially important in determining cancer of the lung, stomach, colon, intestines, kidneys, bladder, bone, brain, etc.

4. *Your physical examination.* One of the outstanding cancer authorities in this country, Dr. George T. Pack, has written:

> "At least 50 percent of all cancers are visible on inspection or within reach of palpation by an examining finger; at least 25 percent more may be seen by the use of special examining instruments inserted within the orifices of the body."

Our diagnostic procedure has been attacked because it does not include biopsy. Medical authorities assert that a positive diagnosis of malignancy can be made only after pathological examination of tissue under a microscope.

Now it is fairly easy to take a sample of tissue from the surface of the body. But to take it from the interior of the body is quite complicated. It can be obtained by an electric snare, or by syringe aspiration; the most common procedure is a surgical operation, in which a sample of tissue is cut out with the scalpel.

Many highly respected medical authorities have opposed biopsies on the grounds that the very act of cutting into cancerous tissue may release malignant cells in the blood stream, bringing about metastases in cases where it has not already occurred. In the end this may cost the patient his life.

For example Dr. C. H. Mayo, the famous surgeon, once wrote in the AMA *Journal* (Vol. 2, p. 213):

> "When they cut out the section and send it away for examination, they have first endangered the person's life through delay; they have next endangered his life through aggravating and stimulating the malignant growth."

A biopsy can verify malignancy and determine its degree, but it will not determine the extent of spread. As a matter of fact, the extent of growth and the spread (metastases) are far more important for prognosis and treatment than the particular grade of cancer presented.

Moreover biopsies are not as reliable as most medical authorities would have us believe. They are as fallible as the doctor who takes them, and the pathologist who reads them. Even when taken by reputable surgeons and analyzed by a competent pathologist, they may be disputed. If negative, it may be proven that the surgeon missed the malignancy by a fraction of an inch. If positive, it may be demonstrated later—after a limb or an important organ has been amputated—that the pathologist's analysis was "in error," the tissue was not malignant after all! This is so common that no pathologist worth his salt will accept as definitive a biopsy report by another pathologist, however brilliant. And conflicting analyses of the same tissue by different pathologists are every-day occurrences.

The result may be tragic. One such instance was related to me recently by a doctor who attended a surgical operation in a well-known New York hospital. A sample of suspect tissue was taken and rushed to the hospital's pathological laboratory. Two pathologists resected it and examined it under the microscope. One said it was definitely malignant, the other declared just as definitely that it was non-malignant. The patient was still on the operating table, so another tissue sample was taken. While the two pathologists were examining it—and still debating—the patient died!

Under pressure to prove to the medical profession that patients treated at the Hoxsey Clinic actually did have cancer, at one time we took samples of tissue from patients and submitted them to AMA-recognized pathological laboratories for analysis. It is noteworthy that in every instance the biopsy report confirmed our clinical diagnosis. This practice ended when the AMA stepped in and forced the pathologists to discontinue their dealings with our clinic. We then employed a qualified pathologist to perform the same work in our own laboratories, only to learn that organized medicine refused to accept our biopsy reports.

With this convincing demonstration that we would never satisfy our medical opponents, no matter what proof we offer, we stopped worrying about biopsies and concentrated on improving other diagnostic techniques.

The fact is, most of our patients already have had biopsies before they come to us for treatment. Moreover we seldom get a case of cancer in its early stages, when diagnosis is particularly difficult. The great majority of our patients are terminal cases who have come to us after long and unsuccessful treatment by conventional methods; by the time we see them the cancer is so far advanced that its symptoms are unmistakable. Another point: the thorough diagnostic procedure outlined earlier usually presents our doctors with enough data to insure a correct diagnosis.

I might add that each of our doctors sees more cases of cancer in a single week than the average practitioner sees in a lifetime. And they are so careful that on numerous occasions patients who have come to us with a diagnosis of cancer by their own doctors have been informed that the latter were mistaken; the patient suffered from chronic colitis, ulcers, non-malignant prostate or rectal conditions, etc.

Thus we finally arrive at the diagnosis in your case. Both diagnosis and prognosis are recorded on your chart. Assuming that we have found cancer, the prognosis depends upon your general condition, the site and type of cancer and the extent of irreparable damage you already have suffered. These same factors (as already stated) determine the exact medication and dosage recommended in your individual case.

The examining doctor frankly discusses our findings with you. If the prognosis is "poor," you may be accepted on a trial basis. This means that you will be given our treatment for a month; at the end of that time you must come back to the clinic for further examination and tests; if you have failed to show any response to the medication, we will then decide whether to continue or drop it.

However, if you decide not to go ahead with our treatment, all you owe us are laboratory fees (which incidentally compare favorably with charges for the same services in any other clinic or laboratory). No charge whatever is made for consultation.

Suppose you decide to take the treatment. If there are cancerous lesions on the surface of your body, you go upstairs to the "external" treating rooms where the powder, salve or clear solutions prescribed in your case is applied. You are also given a prescription for the particular version of our basic internal formula recommended in your case, plus prescriptions for such supportive treatment as may be required. All these prescriptions are filled in our own dispensary. If yours is an internal cancer, you bypass the external treatment and get your supply of internal medication.

The routine outlined here usually takes the better part of two days. When it is completed you go to the business office to discuss the financial arrangements with our business manager or his assistant. *The question of fees is never raised by any of our employees until you are ready to leave.*

You are informed that we do not sell medication; we set a flat fee on the full course of treatment, depending on the severity of your case. In any case our maximum charge is $400, regardless of the length of treatment and the ability or willingness of the patient to pay more. An additional moderate charge is made to cover the cost of laboratory tests and x-ray studies. *Any patient discharged as cured by our clinic is entitled to periodic check-ups without further cost throughout his life.*

Statistics show that the average cancer victim (or his family) spends more than ten times $400 for conventional treatment. Further comment as regards our feé would be superfluous.

If you cannot pay the entire fee we have set at once, you may make arrangements to pay it in monthly installments. If you present a letter from your clergyman, doctor or local authorities stating that you are financially unable to pay anything for treatment, we will treat you without cost. *According to our records approximately 25 percent of all patients treated at this clinic are charity cases.* We never turn away any worthy cancer victim because he (or she) cannot afford treatment.

One of the mischievous lies broadcast about our clinic is that we promise patients we will cure them. Before you leave you will be required to sign the following statement on your case history:

> "It is expressly agreed and understood by the undersigned parties that the Hoxsey Cancer Clinic does not guarantee to cure any ailment or disease for which I may be treated."

No reputable doctor or medical institution will guarantee to cure cancer. We don't have to guarantee a cure; we stand on our record of thousands of cases successfully treated over a period of more than 30 years.

You return to your home and take the medication as prescribed. (There are no provisions for in-patients at our clinic; bed-ridden cases are accommodated at nearby nursing homes and private hospitals.) You will be directed to return to Dallas for further tests, x-ray studies and examination at intervals of one, two or three-month periods depending on your condition.

When do we consider our patients cured?

As a typical external case take H. W. Robbins of Rush Springs, Okla. He first came to our clinic in April 1948 with a large sore on the lower lip. A biopsy taken at that time revealed epidermoid carcinoma Grade 2. Two months after he was put on our treatment the cancer dried up and fell out. Five months later clean scar tissue had entirely filled the hole in his lip. When extensive tests showed no evidence of malignancy he was discharged as "clinically cured." He came back for regular check ups. After three years without a recurrence of the malignancy we considered him cured. At this writing he is still alive and well.

As a typical internal case take Mrs. Laura Bullock of Macon, Georgia. She first came to our clinic in November 1953 with a biopsy report showing cancer of the rectum. Her doctor said it was inoperable. She was having as many as 19 hemorrhages a day, during the preceding year had received a total of 152 blood transfusions, was unable to do any of her household chores. A week after beginning our treatment the hemorrhages ceased; within two weeks she could get around the house without difficulty; within four months she gained 26 lbs. In April 1954, physical examination, laboratory tests and x-rays showed no evidence of cancer anywhere in her system, and we discharged her as "clinically cured." She is directed to come back every year for a check-up. If at the end of five years there has been no recurrence of bleeding, pain or other symptoms of the disease, and she continues to lead a normal life, and our tests fail to turn up any signs of cancer, we will consider her absolutely cured.

Of course we don't cure them all. Many unfortunates come to us after they've undergone maximum surgery (as one patient remarked, *"After a while you run out of lungs!"*) and taken the limit of x-ray or radium. The prognosis by our doctors is "hopeless." We inform the patient of the seriousness of his condition, tell him all that we can hope to do for him is to prevent further extension of the disease and relieve him of pain. If he still insists on taking the treatment, we give it to him—frequently without charge. We do not reject any case, however hopeless, if the patient wishes us to treat him. These are calculated risks, and more often than not we fail to save them.

Frequently patients with "poor" prognoses do not recover. Occasionally a patient with a "fair" prognosis does not respond to our treatment. On the other hand sometimes a patient with a "poor" or even "hopeless" prognosis refuses to die and astounds everyone by making a miraculous recovery.

In all medical history no cure for any disease has ever proven 100 percent effective. We don't contend publicly or privately that ours is. But when our records are finally evaluated we are confident that they will demonstrate that we cure a far greater percentage of cancer—including so-called "terminal cases"—than surgery, x-ray or any other method now known to medical science.

We are not alone in that belief. Nearly every medical man who has visited our clinic, observed our treatment, checked our records and talked with our patients has reached the same conclusion.

Last year a group of ten physicians from all over the nation assembled at our clinic for an independent, impartial investigation of our treatment. They spent two days inspecting the facilities, going over hundreds of case histories and interrogating patients and former patients. On April 12, 1954, they issued a unanimous statement declaring, in part:

"We find as a fact that our investigation has demonstrated to our satisfaction that the Hoxsey Cancer Clinic at Dallas, Texas, is successfully treating pathologically proven cases of cancer, both internal and external, without the use of surgery, radium or x-ray.

"Accepting the standard yardstick of cases that have remained symptom-free in excess of five to six years after treatment, established by medical authorities, we have seen sufficient cases to warrant such a conclusion. Some of those presented before us have been free of symptoms as long as twenty-four years, and the physical evidence indicates that they are all enjoying exceptional health at this time.

"We as a Committee feel that the Hoxsey treatment is superior to such conventional methods of treatment as x-ray, radium, and surgery. We are willing to assist this Clinic in any way possible in bringing this treatment to the American public. We are willing to use it in our office, in our practice on our own patients when, at our discretion, it is deemed necessary.

"The above statement represents the unanimous findings of this Committee. In testimony thereof we hereby attach our signatures."

The names signed to this statement, and the place where each physician practices medicine, are as follows:

S. Edgar Bond, M.D.	Richmond, Indiana
Willard G. Palmer, M.D.	Seattle, Washington
Hans Kalm, M.D.	Aiken, So. Carolina
A. C. Timbs, M.D.	Knoxville, Tennessee
Frederick H. Thurston, M.D., D.O.	Boise, Idaho
E. E. Loffler, M.D.	Spokane, Washington
H. B. Mueller, M.D.	Cleveland, Ohio
R. C. Bowie, M.D.	Fort Morgan, Colorado
Benjamin F. Bowers, M.D.	Ebensburg, Pennsylvania
Roy O. Yeats, M.D.	Hardin, Montana

There is one essential difference between the Hoxsey method and conventional cancer treatments which cannot be demonstrated in the laboratory, brought out by investigation or proven by research. Nevertheless we are sure that it plays an important role in the amazing results obtained at our clinic.

We offer the condemned victim what other doctors deny him: hope, and a fighting chance to conquer the dread disease.

They tell him: *"You are going to die."*

We say: *"You have a chance to live!"*

We are not faith healers. But modern medicine has come to recognize a strong link between the emotional state of a patient and his physical condition. Doctors admit that emotional processes, acting through physical channels, may cause ulcers and even more serious organic disturbances. Psychosomatic medicine holds forth the hope that the emotional processes, if properly channeled, may help a patient to overcome many physical ailments.

Cancer is not only a disease, it is also a psychosis. Tell a victim he is "hopeless" (or let him discover it from his family) and the will to live becomes paralyzed. Show him a way out, strip him of fear and hysteria, give him even a forlorn hope, and the will to live is stimulated. It becomes a powerful ally in the battle against death.

CHAPTER FIVE

Origin of a Cure

I COME of pioneer stock. Lodowick Hoxie, the common ancestor of the numerous Hoxie (as variously spelled) clan in this country, arrived in America about 1650 and settled in the town of Sandwich, in Plymouth Colony. When or where he was born is unknown. His ancestry has been stated variously as Scottish, Welsh, English and Dutch.

The Sandwich records show that in 1657 Lodowick Hoxie was paid three shillings for unspecified services rendered the town. In 1661 he was fined 20 shillings for refusal to assist the town marshal in the execution of his duties, which appears to have been in connection with an attempt by town authorities to destroy the Society of Friends, or Quakers.

It appears that Lodowick became a convert to the Quaker faith. In 1704, when a new Friends meeting place was built, his name is recorded as the individual assigned to "Diet the carpenter, for his share."

His son John Hoxie, born at Sandwich in 1677, moved to Rhode Island and married the daughter of a Quaker preacher. He served as Justice of Westerly, in 1738 was elected town treasurer and overseer of the poor of Charlestown.

Beyond doubt, their Quaker faith had a profound influence upon future generations of the family. The

Friends are a religious fellowship without formal creed or priestly hierarchy; hence the Hoxseys were inclined to reject all religious, political or scientific dogma, to deny the authority of witch-doctors of any kind to impose their theories upon the community as divine doctrine. The Friends are opposed to violence, regard human life as sacred; hence the Hoxsey conviction that the preservation of human life is the duty of all men, not merely the exclusive privilege of those entitled to add "M.D." to their names.

These basic concepts played an important part in the discovery of the Hoxsey method of treating cancer, and in the persistent fight to put that method to work saving lives in spite of opposition, rebuffs and persecution that might have deterred other men.

Our branch of the family remained in Rhode Island for three generations. Shortly after the American Revolution it moved westward with the frontier, first to what is now West Virginia, then to Kentucky, and finally to Madison County, Illinois. There William Hoxsey (as he now spelled his name) and his five sons bought up considerable acreage, built a fine home between Carlinville and Edwardsville, and established one of the finest horse farms in the area.

It was the oldest of those sons, John, who discovered a cure for cancer.

In the Spring of 1840 one of the farm's prize Percherons developed a sore on the right hock. Despite constant treatment the infection grew steadily, encircled the entire hoof, spread to the coronet and then into the fetlock. Exuding pus and a noxious odor, it festered to the bone. The limb became badly swollen, the crippled stallion steadily grew weaker, finally was barely able to limp around the pasture.

"It's cancer," the local vet said. "There's no cure for it. Guess you'll have to shoot him."

But John Hoxsey was loathe to destroy so valuable a stud. He decided to let nature take its course.

That summer an extraordinary thing happened. In June the oozing sore dried and turned black. It seemed to be shrinking. In July cracks appeared at the outer edges, the canker was separating from the healthy surrounding tissue. One day three months later Hoxsey slipped a knife around it and the solid black mass fell out. New scar tissue began to form. By the end of the year the foot was completely healed, the Percheron was sleek and fat again, as good as ever.

What had brought about this miraculous recovery?

Since the first signs of improvement his owner had kept the ailing animal under close observation. He noted that every morning when the stallion was turned out of the stable he made straight for a certain corner of the pasture. Standing knee-deep in a clump of shrubs and flowering plants that grew in profusion there, he would browse contentedly for hours. Hoxsey investigated the clump of vegetation. The plants there looked like ordinary weeds: red clover and alfalfa, buckthorn and prickly ash, as well as a number of others he was unable to identify. One of these, or a combination of them, he reasoned, must be responsible for the amazing cure of the cancer-ridden Percheron.

He picked samples of all the plants growing there, took them to the barn, ground them up with a mortar and began a series of experiments. He mashed the flowers and berries, ground the stalks, boiled the roots. Patiently, month after month, he tried them separately and in various combinations on sick horses in the neighborhood. He studied the ingredients of old home remedies, adding and subtracting them experimentively. Eagerly, week after week, he examined his dumb patients and noted their progress. Finally he hit upon three formulas that proved effective in many cases of cancer.

One was a liquid medicine administered orally.

The second was a salve applied externally to the site of the lesion.

The third was a powder, also applied externally.

John Hoxsey soon acquired quite a reputation in that part of the country as a man with a "healing tetch." From all over Illinois, Indiana and Kentucky breeders brought him horses with "runny neck," fistula, cancer or any persisting open sore. And he cured a large proportion of them.

With native caution, he refused to reveal the secret formulas until, on his death bed, he passed them on to his son.

And that is the story of the origin of the Hoxsey treatment for cancer, as it was related to me by my father who heard it from his father, the son of the man who discovered it.

Fantastic?

An equally fantastic combination of accident and coincidence led to revolutionary discoveries by an ignorant Dutch janitor named Anton van Leeuwenhoek, an eccentric French chemist named Louis Pasteur, an obscure German country doctor named Robert Koch and an unknown Australian nurse named Elizabeth Kenny (to

name a few). Yet their discoveries now are hailed as
landmarks in the history of modern medicine.

John C. Hoxsey, grandson of the founder of the cancer
treatment, was born in Madison County on April 25,
1856. He was my father. The Hoxsey horse farm was a
casualty of the post-Civil War depression. At the age
of 18, soon after his father's death, John Hoxsey took his
patrimony—a string of horses and the secret cancer
formulas—and moved to Bond County. There in 1875
he married Martha Bentley, daughter of a local farmer.
She was of English, Irish and German stock, third generation in this country.

The young couple set up housekeeping on a farm near
Auburn (about 30 miles southwest of the State capital
at Springfield) where my father bred and raised horses.
Up to this time there was no State statue regulating the
practice of medicine. In 1877, when the Illinois Medical
Practices Acts became law, anyone active in the healing
progression for six years could obtain a license. Under
this provision John C. Hoxsey, who had treated horses
for various diseases under the supervision of his father,
was licensed as a veterinary surgeon.

Apparently he inherited the "healing tetch" of his
grandfather. In addition to cancer he was especially skill-
ful in treating fistula and poll evil. Every winter the
Ringling Brothers sent him their ailing circus horses for
treatment. He also developed a successful treatment for
"pink eye" (called "canker eye" in cattle and "lockjaw"
in steers).

In due time twelve children were born to Dr. John
Hoxsey and his wife Martha. I was the youngest; the
date of my birth October 23, 1901. Shortly after my ar-

rival Dad bought a livery stable at Girard, some 10 miles from the farm, and the family moved into town.

Up until the turn of the century Girard had been a sleepy country village with a population of about 1,500, and a quiet square lined with maples and hitching posts. Now great industries were beginning to belch smoke all over the sprawling midwest prairie. To obtain fuel to feed the hungry furnaces, men burrowed deep into the bowels of the Illinois earth, and mountains of raw slag began to deface the landscape, crowding out barns and silos. The towns that once served one of the richest farming communities in the nation underwent a similar transformation. On pleasant summer evenings a horde of husky miners speaking all the diverse tongues of Middle Europe lounged in Girard Square, laughing, jostling, drinking and brawling.

High wages in the nearby mines brought not only an influx of foreign labor, but attracted a flock of vultures; saloons, gambling joints and houses of prostitution.

Such were the scenes of my childhood. And in this sordid and unpromising soil the family formulas for treating cancer sprouted new shoots.

Fired with the notion that a remedy effective in curing horses might be of equal benefit to human beings stricken with the same disease, for some time now my father had been quietly treating cancer patients, first under the supervision of Dr. W. W. Dunton at Sorento (in Bond County) and later under Dr. A. A. Simmons at Girard. His success with these cases led him to open his own office in our home, a block from the Square.

I recall it as a little room with a separate entrance on the street. In one corner was a surgical table for the examination and treatment of patients. Behind this stood a tall cabinet with drawers for instruments and two locked compartments. One held surgical dressings, the other was filled with bottles of cancer medicine, jars of salve and small boxes of cancer powder. Every summer Dad spent several weeks at the farm we still owned near Auburn, concocting a year's supply of medication behind the doors of the barn he'd converted into a laboratory.

From the age of eight on I was entrusted with the key to the cabinet compartment containing the dressings, for it was my duty to see that they were constantly replenished. They were old-fashioned, home-made affairs in a variety of sizes from one to six inches square, and every Saturday afternoon I'd cut enough to last the week from long strips of gauze purchased at the local drug store. Dad trusted no one with the key to the medication compartment; he kept it on his person, day and night.

The first treatment I actually witnessed was that of John Frommie, a prominent local citizen who owned two fine mares bred at our farm. When I first saw him he had a big lump on his neck and another the size of a walnut at the end of his nose. A doctor at Springfield had told him they were cancerous and incurable. I have a vivid memory of his case because I had to prepare a special dressing for him, one that covered the nose and tied behind the ears with four strings. And because after each treatment he would turn to me and demand gruffly:

"Well, son, is my halter ready?"

After six months of treatment the swellings disappeared, and he was discharged as cured. I was a proud boy that day; placing his hand on my head, Mr. Frommie declared:

"Doc, it was Harry and his halters that got me well!"

Right there and then I resolved that when I grew up I would cure people, like my Dad did. I became his constant companion during "office hours" in the early evening, (he attended to his veterinary hospital all day) assisting as best I could in the treatment of patients.

He was pleased with the interest I displayed, and encouraged it. "The boy will make a fine doctor," he frequently observed to my mother. "He has the instinct for it." It was taken for granted that I would go to medical school when I grew up, and become a full-fledged doctor.

Over the course of the next few years hundreds of cancer victims from Girard and neighboring towns came to Dr. Hoxsey for help. One of them was William Hart (everyone called him "Squire" Hart), Justice of Peace at Girard. He had a cancer the size of a silver dollar on the side of his face; the treatment cleared it up in three months. Another prominent patient was Mrs. Lynn Moore, wife of a wealthy local manufacturer. She had a hideous cancer of the breast, was told by eminent specialists that it was incurable. Nevertheless Dad cured her in about eight months, and she outlived many of the physicians who had predicted her early demise.

Results like these broadcast by word of mouth brought more clients and increasing demands on my father's time. Eventually he turned the veterinary hospital over to an assistant and devoted himself almost entirely to the treatment of human cancer.

This involved considerable financial sacrifice. Most of his patients were poor working people and farmers whose meager income barely provided them with a livelihood, let alone the wherewithal for such luxuries as sickness. So his fees were extremely modest—a dollar or two per visit. Moreover, as he never turned anyone away for lack of funds, a large percentage of his practice consisted of charity cases.

"Son," he told me repeatedly, "cancer don't pick and choose. It hits rich and poor, black and white, Catholic, Protestant and Jew. All of them have a right to be treated, whether they can pay for it or not. Healing the sick and saving lives isn't a business, it's a duty and a privilege."

This philosophy wasn't very popular among doctors of his time. Nor, for that matter, is it in vogue in the medical profession today.

Suddenly, late in 1915, occurred an unfortunate accident that changed the entire course of our lives. During a visit to the veterinary hospital my father tripped over a loose board and fell heavily, breaking his nose. Complications set in, he had a long siege of sickness and was unable to take care of his practice. It had taken all he earned to raise a large family; deprived of his earnings, we had to sell the farm and horses to keep our heads above water. The money didn't last very long. My older brothers and sisters were married, had families of their own to support. I decided it was up to me.

At the age of fifteen I quit school and took a job as a "dirt monkey" in the coal mines where my brother Danny worked. Every day, six days a week from 8 A.M. to 6 P.M. I toiled underground, loading an average of eight cars a day, each holding a ton and a half of black mineral. After more than a year of this back-breaking labor my skill in handling animals (acquired on our farm) won me promotion to an easier and better-paying job. I became a "premium mule" driver. Hitching one of the evil tempered but exceptionally strong beasts to four or five carloads of diggers, I would drive it two and a half miles into the pit. Then I'd pick up a train of loaded cars and bring them to the surface. Good "premium mule" drivers were scarce; at the age of seventeen I was earning better than $60 a week, including overtime.

When the mines shut down for the summer I bought a Model-T touring car and ran a taxi service to nearby towns where the lights were brighter, the liquor flowed more freely and the professional ladies were more abundant than in Girard. On the side I sold insurance—home, life, accident, theft, any kind in demand—for a family friend, George Cabareck. Big and husky for my age, I also played professional baseball. During the season I would earn as much as $50 a game pitching ball (under various names) for different small-town teams.

Too busy earning a living to go to school, I knew I needed more education to get into college and become a doctor. So I sent away to the International Correspondence School in Chicago and took a high school correspondence course. Studying hard every night after work, I completed it in three years.

Meanwhile Dad's illness was getting progressively worse. The left side of his face across the nose and under the eye was red and swollen, he ran a constant temperature and suffered severe pain. Finally I persuaded him to consult a specialist in Springfield. The diagnosis was erysipelas (an acute streptococcus infection of the skin). In those days when sulpha drugs and penicillin were still unknown, complications of this disease often proved fatal.

I took my father to St. Louis and Chicago for treatment, but he steadily grew weaker. Just after his 63rd birthday (April 25, 1919) he became completely bedridden.

One afternoon about two weeks later he asked me to go to the People's Bank downtown and bring him his safe deposit box. On the way back I was to stop at the drug store and buy three "Big Chief" writing tablets. I did so. When I brought them to his bedroom he told me to close the door and pull up a chair close to the bed. Hoisting himself to a sitting position with great difficulty, he opened the black steel box, fumbled among deeds and other old family documents, brought out a small white envelope.

"These are the cancer formulas I got from my father and he got from his," he said solemnly. "Now it's my turn to pass them on. I have twelve children and I love you all the same. But when you were just a little shaver, asking questions about my work and watching me treat patients, I knew you had the call to be a doctor. When I got sick you didn't say a word; you just went out and got a job in the mines. You were only a boy, but you did a man's job without complaining. That took guts. After a hard day's work, instead of going out with the boys you kept your nose in books, studying. That showed ambition, and I knew you had what it takes to carry on the good work. That's why I picked you, the youngest, to inherit the family formulas."

Wearied by this long speech, he leaned back on the pillows. I examined the envelope. It was sealed, and outside in his fine copper-plate hand was the inscription: "In the event of my death I want my son Harry to have this." He reached for it, with trembling fingers broke the seal and removed the contents: three small sheets of closely written note paper.

"You won't have to wait until I'm gone to get your inheritance," he said. "I'm going to give it to you now." He handed me one of the "Big Chief" tablets and a pencil. "Now write as I dictate."

Slowly, pausing to rest at frequent intervals, he read the formula for the internal medicine. I copied it down, word for word.

When I had it all, he told me: "Take the tablet into the dining room and write that formula on every page. When you get through, bring it here."

There were 250 blank pages in the tablet. I went right to work. By midnight I had writer's cramp so bad I couldn't hold the pencil, was so groggy that I couldn't see. Lowering my head to my arms, I fell fast asleep. My mother found me there when she got up to fix breakfast. Writing all morning I finally finished and took it in to my father.

He didn't even glance at it. "Do you have it by heart?" he asked. I rattled it off as glibly as my a b c's. Satisfied, he tore the pages to shreds, dropped them into the wastebasket. He did the same with the original. Then he told me to take the basket out and put the paper in the stove, making sure that every scrap was burned. It was a raw wet day, the pot-bellied coal stove in the living room glowed brightly. I dumped the basket and watched the product of hours of hard work go up in smoke.

Back in the bedroom, my father handed me the second "Big Chief" tablet and dictated the formula for the external salve. It lacked a line of filling half a page. "Take it to the dining room and write it twice on every page," he directed. Without a murmur I obeyed. This time I didn't finish until late the following night.

I brought it to my father, recited the formula from memory, disposed of the shreds of paper and received the third and last formula, the one for the external powder. With the end in sight, I put on a burst of speed and wound up my chore that same evening.

Again I had to go through the now familiar ritual of reciting aloud and then destroying the written record. When I returned to the bedroom Dad lay motionless, his eyes shut. I'd never seen him so haggard, so drained. It was as if his mission on earth had ended, now that he'd passed the family responsibilities on to a new generation. Then he opened his eyes, smiled weakly, took my hand. His voice was husky, but surprisingly strong.

"Now you have the power to heal the sick and save lives. What I've managed to do in a tiny part of this state you can do all over the country, all over the world. I've cured a few hundred people; you can cure thousands, tens of thousands.

"But it's not only a gift, son; it's a trust and a great responsibility. Abe Lincoln once said that God must love the common people, because He made so many of them. We're common, ordinary people. No matter how high you go, you must never lose touch with the common people. You must never refuse to treat anybody because he can't pay. Promise me that!"

"I promise," I mumbled.

He smiled sadly, pressed my hand. "I wish I could have done more for you, sent you to college, helped you become a doctor. Now you'll have to go it alone. You've got a long, hard battle ahead, you're going to make yourself a lot of enemies. Many doctors won't like what you're doing because it'll take money out of their pockets. They'll organize against you, fight you tooth and nail, persecute you, slander you, try to drive you off the face of the earth. Don't under-rate them, they're powerful, they're the High Priests of medicine. But in the end you'll win. Because there's one thing they can't do, and that's put back the cancers you removed!"

Exhausted, he closed his eyes. I watched him a long time. When I saw he was asleep, I tiptoed from the room.

A few days later, on May 17, 1919, he died. Dr. W. A. Britten of Virden, Illinois, a family friend who had attended him in his last illness, signed the death certificate which listed the cause of death as erysipelas. We buried him in the Hoxsey family cemetery in Bond County, Illinois.

Dad was right in his prediction of what lay in store for me. However he underestimated the full lengths to which my enemies would go in their efforts to stop me from curing cancer. It never occurred to him that these ghouls would one day dig him up from his grave and vilify his memory.

CHAPTER SIX

Prelude to Battle

Thus, five months before my eighteenth birthday, my destiny was determined for me by a deathbed legacy and a solemn promise to a dying man. I was dedicated to the task of curing cancer.

As a layman I couldn't prescribe an aspirin tablet for a simple headache without getting into trouble. The law was very clear: it's a crime to practice medicine without a license. No matter how many lives I might save, in the eyes of the law I would be a criminal. I could be arrested, fined and sent to jail. And if a patient should die while taking my treatment, even if every doctor in the country previously had given him up as hopeless, I still could be convicted of manslaughter.

I must go to college and medical school, become a full-fledged M.D.—six long years of intensive study, plus one year interneship in a hospital. Then no one could stop me from putting the formulas I'd inherited to work saving the lives of cancer-ridden humanity.

But that took money, and there was precious little left after my father's lengthy illness. Besides, the burden of supporting a widowed mother and sick sister now rested full upon my youthful shoulders.

Somehow, I grimly resolved, I would manage.

With dogged determination I slaved furiously in the coal mines all winter, ran a taxi service all summer, sold insurance on the side and undertook all kinds of odd jobs that brought in added income. Late at night, when everyone else was asleep, I applied myself to my high school correspondence course. Like a miser I counted the pennies and hoarded every dollar we could spare in a cigar box labelled "COLLEGE" hidden in the bottom drawer of the old-fashioned bureau that stood beside my bed.

It was generally known that we had a stock of the cancer remedy under lock and key in the little room that Dad had used as an office, and frequently during the next two years people would come to the house and beg me to treat them. I hated to turn them away, but under the circumstances there was nothing else I could do.

Suddenly tragedy struck again in the Hoxsey household. My sister Bertha, the sickly one, died. A few months later my mother, who'd never fully recovered from Dad's death, also passed on.

Lonely in the big, silent house that once had radiated the warmth and affection of a closely-knit family, I gratefully accepted the invitation of my favorite sister Nora (now Mrs. Walter McClughan) to come live with her and her husband in Taylorville, about 35 miles from Girard. Peabody Mine No. 9 nearby was working full time, and I had no difficulty getting a job there driving a premium mule named "Shorty." My living expenses were small, my personal wants few; more than half my salary every week now went into the cigar box earmarked for college.

Suddenly on the night of Feb. 22, 1921, a wizened old man came into my life and abruptly changed it. He was waiting in the kitchen when I got home from work. His name was S. T. Larkin; he was a citizen of considerable wealth and standing in the community, a retired insurance broker and Civil War veteran. His lower lip and chin were disfigured by a hideous, running sore.

"I've been to three doctors with this," he said, "and they all told me I have cancer, they can't do anything for me, I'll be dead within a year. I knew your daddy well, saw him take sores like this off other people with that medicine of his. I want you to do the same for me."

As many times before in similar cases I carefully explained that I didn't have a license to practice medicine, that it was against the law for me to treat him. He replied:

"Son, when I joined up in '61 and fought to preserve this Union for you and your children and your children's children, they didn't ask me if I had a license to kill rebs. Nobody needs a license to save lives. If I was drowning would you stand by and watch me go down because a sign on yonder tree says 'No Swimming Allowed'?"

There's no adequate answer to that kind of logic and I didn't waste any time trying to find one.

"I'm sorry, Mr. Larkin, but I can't help you," I repeated stubbornly. "I want to go to medical school and get my M.D. so I can set up practice. I can't afford to get into trouble. People will have to wait for treatment until I finish school."

As long as I live I'll never forget his eyes—amazingly bright for such an old man—boring deep into mine, and his solemn rejoinder:

"Son, I can't wait, I'll be dead then. I'm 84 now, have only a few more years to live. But let me tell you, those few years are just as precious to me as a whole lifetime is to you. The first thing they teach doctors is that human life is sacred. You have the power to save mine, if you treat me now. If you don't I'll surely die, and you'll be guilty of murder!"

I knew I was licked. Nothing I could say would make a dent in this remarkable old man's logic. So I finally agreed to treat him, on condition he would keep the treatment a secret.

With mingled feelings of excitement and apprehension I applied the yellow powder to the nasty running sore on his lip and chin, plastered a clean gauze bandage over them—just as I'd seen Dad do hundreds of times in the past—and handed him a big square bottle of the internal tonic to take home with him.

He was my first patient. He'd put his life in my hands. If I failed, I had the law to reckon with. It was an awful responsibility for a 20-year-old boy.

The next time Larkin came in for treatment he was accompanied by E. C. McVicker, a director of the Farmers' National Bank. The banker had an ugly black sore the size of a silver dollar on his temple, near his right ear. A specialist in Springfield had diagnosed it as cancer and informed him that nothing could be done for him. Would I treat him, too?

When I protested that I couldn't take on any more cases, that I must go to college and get a medical degree, he said: "Son, you save my life and I'll give you a check big enough to see you through the best college in the country!"

I hesitated, then shrugged: "Might as well treat two as one." So I took on my second patient. He too was sworn to silence.

A few weeks later when I got home from work I found

the two of them waiting for me. With them was J. Cal Hunter, a wealthy retired farmer whose son Wayne led the high-school band that played at local concerts. The elder Hunter's right hand was bandaged. Unravelling the gauze, he revealed a sickening sight. The entire back of his hand was a mass of rotting flesh, the rest of it was baked as if in an oven. He told me it started with a small lesion which a local doctor had diagnosed as cancer. Intensive x-ray treatment badly burned the hand, but failed to halt the spread of the malignancy. Perhaps I could help him.

Before I could muster up my usual excuses Larkin, a mischievous glint in his eyes, drawled: "Might as well treat three as two!"

I flared up. "It's no joke. Hell, I can't even put a shin plaster on my mule Shorty without running afoul of the law! If one of you dies I get the blame, and maybe spend the rest of my life in the hoosegow. If you get well you'll blab it all over the county, and I'll wind up in jail for practicing medicine without a license. No matter how it turns out, I'm in trouble."

Tall, dignified McVicker put his arm around me.

"It's no joke to us either," he said soberly. "Each of us is fighting for his life. We've come to you looking for a miracle. You're our last hope. Take it from me, it's God's work you're doing, and as long as you do that no harm can come to you. If anyone tries to make trouble we'll stand by you, come Hell or high water. That's a promise!"

So now I had three patients. By this time I knew it was useless to bind them to silence. If they got well their friends and their friends' friends too would hear about it; those with cancer would beat a path to my door. And I'd have to treat them all, regardless of the consequences.

Sure enough during the next few months, as the putrescent sores disappeared from Larkin's face, McVickers' temple and Hunter's hand, I was besieged by unfortunates who begged me to do the same for them. Soon I had so many patients under treatment that I had to give up my job in the coal mine to take care of them.

Among those I treated during this period were Russell Price, a cigar manufacturer of Taylorville; B. E. Bulpitt, the local undertaker; Mrs. T. J. Black, wife of a lumber mill operator; Mrs. Charles Sleighbough, wife of the town's leading jeweler; Fred Auchenbach, vice-president and cashier of the Taylorville National Bank.

All of them had been told by their own doctor that they had cancer. And they all recovered after taking my treatment.

Perhaps the most spectacular case of all was that of Mrs. H. E. Stroud, 45-year-old wife of a nearby farmer. In September 1923—five months before I first met her—Dr. Nelms of Taylorville informed her that she had cancer of the left breast and sent her to the hospital at Springfield to have it removed. There she was told it was too late for surgery; the disease had metastasized to the glands under the arm. They packed the breast with radium, gave her a total of 10 hours of deep x-ray treatment, finally informed her husband that nothing further could be done, she was incurable.

Bulpitt the undertaker (whom I'd treated for cancer of the mouth) drove me over to the Stroud farm one Sunday. Entering the door the characteristic odor of decaying flesh almost knocked me off my feet. The emaciated

patient (she weighed only about 75 lbs. now) was a pitiful sight; the cancer had eaten away her entire breast,
broken out in numerous places on her body.

Taking her husband aside, I told him: "There's nothing I can do for her; she's too far gone. There isn't
a chance in a million that she'll get well." With tears in
his eyes he begged me to try, and I finally yielded.

To everybody's amazement (including my own) after
a few treatments she began to improve, eventually made
a recovery that was little short of miraculous. She's still
alive today, at the age of 75. Her son, the Rev. Fred
Stroud, who now occupies a pulpit at Nashville, Tenn.,
has recommended numerous patients to my clinic in
Dallas.

When I took on Mrs. Stroud I promised myself that
she would be my last patient as an unlicensed healer.
Although I'd had exceptional luck so far—not one of the
people I'd treated had died—I had a premonition that
the law of averages soon would catch up with me. Moreover, never losing sight of my plan to become a doctor,
I now had saved up enough money to see me through
college and medical school.

The problem was to find a college with a good pre-
med course that would accept my mail-order high school
diploma. I had nowhere to turn for advice; for obvious
reasons I wasn't on good terms with any of the local doctors. At this point my good friend Louis Hirschberg, an
auctioneer, came up with a solution. He took me to Chicago and introduced me to Dr. Maximilian Meinhardt,
an eye-ear-nose specialist and head of a large sanitarium.

Dr. Meinhardt, it turned out, was far more interested
in my method of treating cancer than in helping me get

into medical school. "You have seven months before the Fall term begins," he said. "Meanwhile I'd like to see if your cancer remedy really works. Would you be willing to treat a few patients under my supervision at this sanitarium?"

Sensing a challenge, I immediately accepted. Dr. Meinhardt passed the word among his colleagues that he wanted some cancer cases to treat, and within a few weeks we had ten patients at his sanitarium under my care. Their doctors, skeptical at the onset of our little experiment, were amazed as time went on and their patients began to show definite signs of improvement.

One day I overheard one of these physicians, Dr. Bruce Miller, remark: "Even if all these cases react favorably, it still isn't proof that this treatment is effective. The question is, how many of them will be alive a year, two years or five years from now?"

I replied quickly: "You can find out by talking with patients I treated at Taylorville, and with those treated by my father at Girard."

"I think I'll do just that, young fellow," he retorted, with a friendly smile.

At that time I was commuting between Chicago and Taylorville, where I still had some patients under treatment. Dr. Miller accompanied me on my next trip home. He spent several days interviewing Larkin, McVickers, Auchenbach and other people I'd treated, and he conferred with their doctors. I also took him to see Mrs. Stroud, then in the second month of treatment. Examining her, he said gravely:

"If you cure her, my boy, you can cure any cancer case on earth!"

"She's going to get well," I asserted confidently. "You should have seen her when my treatment began."

The following week, on my return to Chicago, I received a telephone call from Dr. Miller asking me to call at his office. As soon as I finished caring for my patients at the sanitarium I went to see him. He told me he'd just come back from Girard, where he'd investigated several of the cases treated by my father.

"In more than 30 years of practice I've never seen or heard anything like this," he declared. "By all the laws of medicine most if not all of those people should be dead and buried long ago. Yet they seem to be in perfect health, without a trace of cancer so far as I can ascertain. It's incredible! If I hadn't seen them with my own eyes, heard their stories with my own ears and had them confirmed by their own doctors I wouldn't believe it!"

Observing my triumphant smile, he said with deliberation:

"Where the human body is concerned, we doctors like to foster the myth that modern medicine is omniscient. We have to, it's our stock in trade. Otherwise people wouldn't place their bodies and lives in our hands, we'd starve to death. To the average person his body is a divine mystery and the physician a high priest, an oracle who alone can unravel its meaning. Sometimes we doctors get so's we believe that myth ourselves.

"Unfortunately it isn't true. We *do* know a lot about the general structure of the human body and the functions of some of its principal organs. We are trained to observe symptoms and to reason out the pathological disturbances that may cause them. We know a few medicines that will cure a few specific ailments. We can set bones, perform surgery. And that's more than laymen can do.

"However volumes could be written about what we don't know, even about the most fundamental facts of life. For example, we know next to nothing about the essential trigger-mechanism of life and death. We don't know why women menstruate, how the fertilized egg reaches the tube, why it takes precisely nine months for a child to be born. We don't know what causes the heart to beat and what causes it to stop beating. We don't know where blood is made, what causes cells and bones to renew themselves, why the lungs work as they do, how the kidneys secrete urine. Oh, we have all kinds of theories. But we don't *know*.

"One of the things we know very little about is cancer. We don't know what causes it, why normal cells suddenly flare up and go on a rampage. We don't know how to stop their wild propagation, nor how to prevent them from spreading through the body, except possibly in the primary stages of the disease when we can cut or burn them out. Any sincere doctor will admit that surgery, radium and x-ray are useless once the disease has metastasized. We're groping around for a more effective treatment. Thus far we haven't found it."

He paused, his eyes probing mine, then continued:

"The point I'm making is this: we can't permit an un-initiated layman like you to come up with a solution to a medical problem that has baffled the best scientific minds for thousands of years. If we did, public confidence in the omniscience of the priesthood would be undermined, our privileged status—and our incomes—would be threatened. You'll find damn few doctors with the independence, honesty and courage to admit you can cure cancer. They don't dare. If they did, organized medicine would close its ranks in mutual protection and freeze them out. They'd lose their licenses, be hounded out of the profession."

I asserted confidently: "Well, in that case the answer is simple. I'll go to medical school and become a doctor, and put the treatment on a scientific basis."

Then the bombshell fell. Slowly shaking his head, Dr. Miller stated flatly:

"You don't stand a chance, you'll never get in. I've made inquiries, talked with doctors in Taylorville and Girard. They're out to get you. They've already complained to the State Board that you're practicing medicine without a license, promoting a 'fake' cancer cure. An investigator has been sent down from Springfield and as soon as he gets enough evidence a warrant for your arrest will be issued. You're blackballed, no medical school will let you in the door."

Numb with shock, I just sat there and stared at him. "How can they keep me from going to school?" I demanded incredulously.

Dr. Miller said wearily: "Few outsiders seem to realize that the medical profession in this country has been organized into a closely-knit association whose primary concern is the protection and benefit of its members. It sets the standards for medical schools all over the country and issues lists of hospitals approved for internship. Thus it is able to regulate the supply of new doctors, and when necessary to keep 'undesirables' out of the profession.

"You come under that heading. You're 'undesirable'

because you're practicing the sacred art of healing without the proper credentials. They can't keep you from going to college, but they can and will see to it that no recognized medical school will accept you as a student. And they'll make damned sure you never get a license to practice medicine anywhere in this country."

All my fine plans collapsing into a heap of rubble, I cried desperately: "What do I do now?"

He arose, began to pace up and down the room.

"Many doctors don't like what's happening to the medical profession these days," he said abruptly. "Some of us are old-fashioned enough to believe that our first duty is to our patients, not to our purses. We've gone along with the organization because we have to; if we didn't, other doctors wouldn't refer patients to us, we wouldn't be permitted to practice in many hospitals.

"However since my experience in Taylorville and Girard I've been wrestling with my conscience. I'm convinced that your treatment is effective in combatting some—if not all—types of cancer, that it's far superior to any other treatment now being used and should be made available to cancer sufferers at once. And I've decided that it's my duty to help you do that.

"I have a degree from the College of Physicians and Surgeons in Chicago and I'm licensed to practice medicine in this State. No one can dispute my right to treat cancer or any other disease.

"Now I'm willing to go to Taylorville and join you in opening a clinic where your method will be exclusively employed. I'll be the medical director of the clinic; you'll be my assistant, a technician, applying the treatment under my direction. If after a year or two we can produce hundreds of cancer cases successfully treated under proper medical supervision, the profession will have to acknowledge that the treatment we use is an effective cure for cancer!"

I told him I'd have to give his proposition some thought, and left. On my return to Taylorville I discussed the whole situation at length with Fred Auchenbach and the president of his bank, Troy Long. In their opinion this was the only logical solution to my predicament. And they assured me that their bank would back me to the limit in setting up the proposed clinic.

So a few days later a 57-year-old physician with a conscience and a 23-year-old ex-coal miner determined to carry out his assigned mission in life sat down together and mapped out ambitious plans to demonstrate to the world that cancer can be cured without the use of surgery, x-ray or radium.

We agreed to form a partnership. Dr. Miller, as medical director of the clinic, would examine and diagnose all patients and build up a solid bulk of case histories in accordance with the highest medical standards. My job was that of a technician; I was to provide the medication and administer it under his supervision.

We agreed I would not have to divulge the secret formulas I'd inherited until such time as they would be recognized as a valid contribution to medical practice. Then we would make them available to the entire profession without fee or financial return.

We agreed not to charge more than $300 for the full treatment. Except that, in accordance with my promise to my father, nobody would be turned away for lack of funds. If a patient was unable to pay, he would be treated free of charge.

Dr. Miller volunteered to move his medical library to Taylorville.

"You already have as much practical experience with cancer as the average M.D. gets in a lifetime," he said. "A knowledge of medical theory will be of considerable value. As we go along I'll teach you all I know, the rest you can get from books. And you can keep abreast of the latest experiments in the field by reading current medical publications which I receive."

That suited me fine. Because I still hoped that one day the "crime" I committed in curing cancer without a license would be vindicated by results obtained in the new clinic, I would be permitted to enter medical school and become an accepted practitioner. And I was determined to keep up my studies.

On March 1, 1924 we opened our clinic in a house we'd rented for that purpose at 401 Park Street in Taylorville. Almost immediately we were swamped with patients.

Dr. Miller was a scrupulously thorough practitioner and his professional competence made a profound impression on everyone. He questioned each patient lengthily until he had a complete medical history including earlier ailments, current symptoms, previous diagnosis, prognosis and treatment. Refusing to accept any diagnosis of cancer—even when accompanied by a biopsy report—as infallible, he insisted on verifying it by personal examination. We were not equipped for extensive laboratory tests, but if there was any doubt in his mind as to the proper verdict he would invariably insist that the patient go to a recognized laboratory for the proper tests.

"Unfortunately," he would say, "most general practitioners lack the necessary knowledge and experience for accurate diagnosis in cases of this sort. As a result they either treat the poor devil for everything under the sun except cancer, or they scare him to death by diagnosing cancer where none exists.

"In this clinic we can't afford to make mistakes. Other doctors bury theirs and none is the wiser. Even if another doctor finds out, he is bound to silence by the rigid code of professional ethics. But they'll dig ours up and beat us to death with them, if they can."

Thus partly by absorption—watching and listening to Dr. Miller—partly by treating patients under his exacting eye and partly by assiduous study of the texts he recommended, I served my medical apprenticeship and perfected the techniques acquired earlier in the art of healing cancer.

News of the clinic spread rapidly, patients flocked in from as far as 200 miles away. Within two months they were sitting in each other's lap, the small premises we occupied no longer would accommodate them all, we were forced to seek larger quarters.

CHAPTER SEVEN

First Clash with the AMA

One of the landmarks of Taylorville was the three-story converted residence on Main Street occupied by the local Loyal Order of Moose. My friend and former patient Fred Auchenbach, an official of the Lodge, informed us that the board of trustees might be induced to sell the property if persuaded that it would be employed for a worthy purpose. There was plenty of room not only for our rapidly-expanding clinic, but for a 25-bed hospital. He said his bank would finance the entire transaction.

Accordingly one Sunday afternoon in March, accompanied by Dr. Miller, I appeared before a meeting of the membership in the auditorium of the Lodge and presented our proposal. To reinforce my arguments nearly a dozen of my cured patients were present including Larkin, McVicker, Hunter, Bulpitt, Mrs. Sleighbough, Mrs. Stroud and Fred Baugh, secretary of the Lodge. After hearing their testimony the members voted unanimously to sell us the building.

At this point a stranger in the audience demanded the floor. He identified himself as Lucius O. V. Everhard, an insurance broker and member of a Moose Lodge in Chicago. He said he'd recently written a large policy on the life of Dr. Malcolm L. Harris, chief surgeon at the Alexian Brothers and the Henrotin Memorial hospitals in

Chicago, and a power in the American Medical Association (he later became its President).

"If half of what I've heard today is true," Everhard declared, "Taylorville is too small to hold this clinic. Cancer is a national calamity. If Hoxsey is willing I'll telephone Dr. Harris and try to get his support for a clinic in Chicago, where the Hoxsey treatment can reach a wider audience."

I was more than willing, I was excited and elated. Here was the answer to all my problems. With the backing of Dr. Harris, medical recognition of the Hoxsey treatment was a foregone conclusion. Moreover his recommendation would be an "Open, Sesame" to any medical school in the country.

Everhard immediately put through a long-distance call, reached the eminent AMA official at his home, poured out what he'd just seen and heard, urged that Dr. Miller and I be permitted to demonstrate our treatment on patients at one of the Chicago hospitals. There was a pause, then came the reply:

"Have them meet me tomorrow morning at 8:30 at the south door of the Alexian Brothers Hospital!"

The distance from Taylorville to Chicago by road is more than 200 miles. Setting out in my car immediately after dinner that same night Everhard, Dr. Miller and I arrived at our destination just before midnight. We checked into the Sherman Hotel. Bright and early next morning we were waiting outside the hospital.

Promptly at 8:25 a shiny black Locomobile piloted by a chauffeur drew up at the door and Dr. Harris alighted. He was a thin, slightly-built gentleman (about 5 feet 6 inches tall) in his late fifties with steel-grey hair and a small, closely-cropped mustache. Well dressed and carefully groomed, he moved with the dignity and self-assurance of a man of distinction. As he gave me a limp hand and inspected me from head to foot I was painfully conscious of my rough, calloused miner's paws and ill-fitting store clothes, my Sunday best. Leading the way into the hospital, he said:

"I have a patient I want you to see. Frankly, he's a terminal case. We've done all we can for him, so there's no harm in experimenting. I don't expect you to cure him. But if your treatment produces no unfavorable reaction, we'll go ahead and try it on other cases not so far advanced."

That sounded fair enough. We took the elevator to the third floor where we were met by Dr. Daniel Murphy, the resident in charge. After a brief conference with Dr. Harris he took us to the room where the patient lay.

Thomas Mannix, 66-year-old former desk sergeant at the Sheffield Avenue Police Station, seemed more dead than alive. His cadaverous appearance was enhanced by a head completely bald except for a fringe of grey hair, sunken orbs, long sharp nose and grizzled mustache over a bony chin. The mottled skin hung loosely from his scrawny neck, his once-burly frame had shrunk to little more than 70 lbs. The chart at the foot of his bed showed that a prodigious amount of morphine was being administered at regular intervals to dull his pain. Unfastening the patient's gown, Dr. Murphy drew it away from the left shoulder and disclosed a hideous mass of diseased flesh about six inches in diameter. It was seared and baked by intensive x-ray treatment which had, however, failed to halt the progress of the disease.

After a minute examination of the patient, Dr. Miller drew me aside and told me that in his opinion there wasn't a ghost of a chance that Mannix would survive our treatment. I was less pessimistic. Bending over the bed, I said with deep conviction:

"Sarge, if you help us we'll pull you through. You can get well. It depends on how hard you fight. Do you understand me?"

He was too weak to reply verbally, but I was sure I detected a responsive flicker in his dull, faded eyes.

Dr. Harris and Dr. Murphy watched intently as I applied a thick coating of the yellow powder to the gaping lesion, and Dr. Miller put a dressing over it. We left a bottle of our internal medicine with directions that the patient receive a teaspoonful three times per day, and advised the two doctors that we would be back in a week to administer another treatment.

On our way back to Taylorville, Dr. Miller observed: "If we pull this one through, it'll be a miracle!"

I patted his arm. "Don't worry, Doc. Mrs. Stroud looked even worse when I first saw her, and she recovered. We've given Mannix hope, he'll fight for his life now. And that's half the battle."

My confidence was justified in full.

Within two weeks the surface of the pustulant sore turned black and started to dry, a sure sign that our medicine was working on the malignancy.

Within four weeks a hard crust had formed, the cancer was shrinking and pulling away at the edges from the normal tissue. Moreover the rapid improvement in the patient's general physical condition amazed all who saw him. He was able to sit up now, his eyes were bright and alert and the pain had vanished, he no longer needed morphine to sustain him, his appetite had returned, he was beginning to pick up weight.

Two weeks later he was walking around, taking care of his physical needs, champing at the bit and impatient to get back to work. When he saw us he chortled:

"I guess we fooled 'em, didn't we, Doc? Can't wait to get back to the station house and see the look on the faces of the boys. They was all set to give me an Inspector's funeral."

His daughter Kate Mannix, a registered nurse who had assisted in the care of her father, stopped us in the corridor to express the gratitude of the family.

"We feel just as if he's been raised from the dead," she declared. "We'd given up hope. Anyone who's seen a loved one dying of cancer will know what a nightmare we've been through. Now we're just about the happiest people on earth. We'll remember you in all our prayers. And if there's any other way we can show our appreciation, please let us know."

To me these simple, heartfelt words were the richest reward any man could ask.

That same day we informed Dr. Harris that necrosis of the cancerous mass in the policeman's shoulder was complete, it had separated from the normal tissue and could be lifted out within two days. He could scarcely believe his ears, insisted on examining the patient himself.

"This is something I want every doctor in the hospital to witness," he asserted. "Would you be willing to perform that operation in the amphitheatre before the entire staff?"

Dr. Miller and I welcomed the opportunity.

That Wednesday at 10 A.M. when we arrived at the amphitheatre of the Alexian Brothers Hospital we found it buzzing with excitement. The gallery of seats surrounding the operating pit was crowded with more than 60 internes, house physicians and visiting doctors. Scrubbed and gowned, we took up our positions in the pit beside Dr. Harris. He cleared his throat, and the gallery suddenly was silent.

He began with a concise review of the case, detailed the various treatments given the patient, described the latter's condition when he was turned over to us. Then he introduced us and explained our procedure. When he'd finished the patient was wheeled in and we took over.

Dr. Miller removed the bandages from Mannix' shoulder. Self-conscious and tense with awareness that scores of trained eyes were following every move under the bright operating light, I picked up the forceps, scraped and probed the black mass of necrosed tissue. It moved freely at the perimeter but was still anchored at the base. I worked it loose, lifted it out with the forceps, deposited it on the white enamel tray provided for that purpose. And that's all there was to the operation.

Dr. Harris inspected the cavity left by the tumor. There was no sign of blood, pus or abnormal tissue, clean scar tissue already had begun to form. "In time it will heal level with the surrounding flesh," I told him. "There will be no need for plastic surgery."

Shaking his head incredulously, he declared: "It's amazing, if I hadn't seen it I wouldn't believe it!"

Then, looking closer: "What about the necrosis in the clavicular bone?"

"That was caused by x-ray. It too will slough off."

Doctors and internes filled the pit and crowded around the operating table, inspecting the patient, examining the necrosed tissue, firing questions at Dr. Miller and me. The entire demonstration had taken less than half an hour but it was nearly noon before we could break away. Dr. Harris accompanied us to the door and asked where we were stopping.

I told him I was at the Sherman Hotel, would remain there a couple of days before returning to Taylorville. He promised to get in touch with us before we left. On our way back to the hotel I was jubilant.

"We did it! Now they'll have to admit that we have a treatment that cures cancer!"

Dr. Miller smiled skeptically. "It's not that easy. Wait until Harris gets a chance to think it over and discusses it with other doctors. They'll come up with all kinds of reasons why our treatment wasn't responsible for the patient's recovery. There's more at stake here than you think—prestige, and money, millions invested in x-ray and radium equipment. . . ."

At that time it sounded fantastic, and I quickly changed the subject.

Early next morning I was awakened by a telephone call from Dr. Harris. "I'd like to have a talk with you," he said. "I'm at my office in the Field Annex, about two blocks from your hotel. Can you come right over?"

Glancing at my watch, I discovered that it was just 7:15 A.M. I agreed to meet him in half an hour. Hastily I showered, shaved, threw on my clothes and—postponing breakfast—set off to keep the appointment.

Dr. Harris occupied an extensive suite on the seventh floor of the imposing office building. Bristling with early morning energy he met me at the door, ushered me into his private office, motioned me into a chair beside his desk. Surveying me appraisingly, he began:

"Hoxsey, the demonstration you put on yesterday has opened up an entirely new vista in the treatment of cancer. I spent most of last evening discussing the Mannix case with some of my colleagues, and they agree that his amazing recovery is convincing evidence that chemical compounds such as you use offer the best hope to eradicate this disease. It's not just the yellow powder you used; that I suppose is an escharotic. It's the amazing improvement in his general condition as the result of the medicine you've been giving him."

This was it, the official recognition I'd been seeking so avidly. Giddy with triumph, I could scarcely control an impulse to jump up and gratefully shake his hand.

"Of course," he cautioned, "it's much too early to say that Mannix is cured of cancer. There may be a recurrence; we'll have to wait five years or more before we can reach a definite conclusion. Moreover we can't be sure that your treatment actually cures cancer until we've tried it out on hundreds of other patients and thus can evaluate its effectiveness."

I broke in eagerly: "We can show you hundreds of people who've already taken our treatment and been cured!"

He shook his head impatiently. "That's not scientific proof. We must set up a large-scale experiment under absolute medical controls. Our doctors must select the cases treated so that we're treating cancer; they must administer the treatment in order to determine the effective dosage, unfavorable reactions etc.; the patients must be kept under constant medical observation to ward off the possibility that some other factor may account for their recovery. It's a long-range project involving technical skill, hard work and considerable expense."

He paused significantly.

"Dr. Harris," I assured him fervently, "I'll cooperate 100 percent in any experiments you care to make with the Hoxsey treatment. All I want is the opportunity to prove that it actually cures cancer, and is made available as widely as possible to relieve human suffering."

He nodded approvingly. Opening a drawer in his desk he produced a sheaf of papers fastened together with a clip and handed it to me. "I was sure you'd feel that way about it, so I had my lawyers draw up a contract. Read it, sign it and we'll get busy at once in setting up an organization to handle the experiments."

There were ten double-spaced, typewritten, legal sized sheets in the contract. I read slowly, struggling with the involved, unfamiliar legal terms. Dr. Harris arose and strolled over to the window, contemplating the vast expanse of Lake Michigan in the distance.

By the time I reached the bottom of the second page I discovered that I was to turn over all the formulas of the Hoxsey treatment to Dr. Harris and his associates, and relinquish all claims to them. They would become the personal property of the doctors named in the contract.

On the following page it specified that I was to mix and deliver 10 barrels of the internal medicine, 50 lbs. of the powder and 100 lbs. of the yellow ointment, and instruct a representative of the doctors in the method of mixing these compounds.

Farther along I agreed to close my cancer clinic and henceforth take no active part in the treatment of cancer.

My reward for all this was set forth on next to the last page. It appeared that during a ten-year experimental period I would receive no financial remuneration. After that I was to get 10 percent of the net profits. Dr. Harris and his associates would set the fees—and collect 90 percent of the proceeds.

Stunned and appalled by this incredible document, I turned back and reread the principal clauses to make sure my eyes weren't playing me tricks. There it was, all neatly typed in black and white. The eminent doctor turned away from the window, seated himself behind his desk and favored me with a nonchalant smile.

"Well," he said heartily, "I trust it's all clear to you."

It was all too clear. He and his friends were trying to trick me out of the family formulas, abscond with the fame and prestige attached to the discovery of a real cure for cancer, and thereby enrich themselves fabulously at my expense—and the expense of millions of helpless cancer victims. Disillusioned and angry, I could scarcely speak. Finally I found my voice.

"Before signing this," I said carefully, "I'd like to show it to a lawyer. Mr. Samuel Shaw Parks, who has offices in the Delaware Building on Randolph Street, was my father's attorney. I'll consult him and be guided by his advice. Perhaps he'll suggest some changes. . . ."

Dr. Harris' smile turned frosty. "There won't be any changes," he snapped. "We've set forth the only conditions under which your treatment can be ethically established. Unless you accept them in their entirety, no reputable doctor will have anything to do with you or your treatment."

With considerable effort I kept a tight rein on my temper. He has a powerful organization behind him, I kept telling myself. You mustn't antagonize him.

"In any case, I'll have to have some time to think over your proposition." I stood up.

His eyes, friendly as a cobra's, took my full measure. "Hoxsey," he said levelly, "until you sign that contract you can't see Sgt. Mannix again."

He picked up the telephone, called the hospital, asked for the superintendent, Brother Anthony. "This is Dr. Harris. Until further orders, neither Hoxsey nor Dr. Miller are to be admitted to your hospital, or to communicate in any way with the patient Thomas Mannix."

I waited until he hung up the receiver, then seized the telephone and called the Mannix home. Before I could be connected Dr. Harris reached over the desk and tried to take the telephone away from me. My left elbow flipped up, caught him squarely in the chest and sent him flying into his chair. It promptly toppled over, depositing him in a most undignified position on the floor.

Miss Mannix came on the wire and I explained the situation to her. "If you want your father to get well you'd better get him out of the hospital and take him home. I'll be over to see him this evening and change the dressing."

She assured me she'd get him home immediately.

Dr. Harris picked himself off the floor, his dignity considerably ruffled, his face as red as a boiled lobster.

"You'll never get away with this!" he shrilled. "If you as much as touch that patient I'll have you arrested for practicing medicine without a license. As long as you live you'll never treat cancer again. We'll close down your clinic, run you and that quack doctor of yours out of Illinois. Try and set up anywhere else in this country and you'll wind up in jail."

Without bothering to reply I walked out.

Returning to the hotel, I received a telephone call from Dr. Miller. He was in a booth across the street from the Alexian Brothers Hospital, where he'd gone to see our patient. They'd refused to let him in. I explained what had happened at Dr. Harris' office. When I finished, there was a long silence. Finally he sighed:

"Well, that does it. Harris won't rest now until he's put us out of business. You've made yourself a powerful enemy. It's not just a few local doctors you have to reckon with now, it's the whole Medical Association. They'll hound you and blacken your name, and that of everyone associated with you, from one end of the country to the other. You're young and brash, but how long do you think you can go on bucking the entire medical profession?"

I didn't hesitate a moment. "Until I prove to the world that I can cure cancer. As my Daddy once told me, there's one thing doctors can't do, and that's put back the cancers we remove. Don't worry about me, Doc; I can take anything they dish out. How about you?"

His voice came back strong over the wire: "I still say a doctor's first duty is to his patients. I'll string along with you, my boy."

He waited outside while Kate Mannix, over the strenuous objection of hospital authorities, signed her father out of the institution. When they finally emerged he helped them into a cab and escorted them home. There we continued to treat the policeman until he was fully recovered, three months later.

Thomas Mannix eventually returned to duty at the Sheffield Avenue police station, where he served as desk sergeant until he was retired on pension. There was no recurrence of cancer. He died ten years later. The cause of his death: *Coronary sclerosis.* I have a copy of his death certificate before me now, and it does not mention cancer.

Does this story sound fantastic?

In his book ORIGIN OF A CURE Dr. William F. Koch relates that his troubles with the AMA began when he refused to assign all rights to his cancer treatment to a syndicate of officials of the Wayne County (Mich.) Medical Society. And there is convincing evidence (see Chapter 18) that AMA opposition to the cancer drug *krebiozen* followed close on the heels of refusal by its discoverers to sell their rights to the Secretary of the AMA, acting on behalf of a leading pharmaceutical house.

Is it possible to believe that highly respected medical authorities, for personal profit or otherwise, would willfully doom millions of human beings to death by arbitrarily withholding treatment that could save them?

Let's take a close look at the American Medical Association, its history and its activities.

CHAPTER EIGHT

The High Priests of Medicine

On MAY 5, 1847, a conclave of 255 eminent physicians representing the medical talent of 28 states assembled in Philadelphia to midwife the birth of a national organization "*to supply more efficient means than have been hitherto available . . . for exciting and encouraging emoluments and concert of action in the profession.*" The delivery was normal, and after considerable discussion the newborn babe was proudly christened The American Medical Association.

A rather puny and ineffectual child, perennially ailing and on the point of death, the Association managed to struggle along for 50 years without attracting much attention or accomplishing anything of significance. At the beginning of this century it could count no more than 9,000 members among the 100,000 regular practicing physicians in the U.S.

About that time three astute medico-politicians decided to take over the moribund organization, revitalize it, and convert it into a machine for the conquest of power far beyond the wildest dreams of its founders.

The sparkplug of this ambitious enterprise was a Dr. George Henry Simmons of Lincoln, Nebraska. According to his official biography he was born in Moreton, England on Jan. 2, 1852; migrated to this country at the age of 18; attended Tabor College and the University of Nebraska;

obtained his M.D. from Hahnemann Medical College (a homeopathic institution) in 1882; secured a "regular" M.D. from Rush Medical College in 1892.

Investigators put on his trail later came up with an entirely different story. They charged he'd never graduated from college and didn't have a medical degree when he hung out his shingle and began the practice of medicine. He actively practiced for 10 years, they asserted, before making it nice and legal by getting a mail-order diploma from Chicago. He apparently did it without missing a day's work at Lincoln—more than 500 miles away. A remarkable feat!

It is a matter of public record that during the 1880s "Doc" Simmons advertised extensively in local newspapers as a "Homeopathic Physician" and "Specialist in Diseases of Women." The ads stated that he'd *spent a year and a half in the largest hospitals of London and Vienna*" and held a diploma as "Licentiate of Gynecology and Obstetrics" from the Rotunda Hospitals in Dublin, Ireland.

There is no evidence that any of his claims was true.

Many of his ads (see reproduction on p. 150k) also carried the significant notation "*A limited number of lady patients can be accommodated at my residence*"—in those days the typical come-on of an abortionist and quack in venereal disease. At one time, in partnership with two other doctors, he operated a "Lincoln Medical Institute" which blatantly advertised, among other things, a humbug "Massage and Movement Cure" and an equally fake "Compound Oxygen" treatment.

Dr. Olin West, Secretary of the AMA, was asked to explain these ads when he appeared before a U.S. Senate investigating committee in 1930. He reluctantly admitted they were unethical and smacked of quackery, declared that if any doctor now were to advertise in such fashion *"we would oppose it, expose it and condemn it"* and kick the offender out of organized medicine.

None of these nasty things ever happened to "Doc" Simmons. On the contrary. After serving several years as secretary of the Nebraska State Medical Society and editor of the *Western Medical Review,* in 1898 he wangled a job as editor of the AMA *Journal* at the munificent salary of $5,000 per year.

Moving to Chicago to devote full time to his new duties, he found the Association in a sad state of decay, decrepitude and insolvency. A single rented room served both as headquarters of the organization and editorial rooms of its official publication. The only other salaried employe, the Secretary of the Association, was totally incompetent; the organization itself was torn by dissension, drifting along without direction or purpose; the *Journal* was dull and uninteresting, largely given over to paid testimonials for worthless nostrums and proprietary remedies.

Simmons set to work to clean house. A shrewd politician and promoter, within three months he managed to ease out the bewildered Secretary and annex that job to the one he already held.

Meanwhile an ambitious plan was percolating in his brain. This was an era of Big Business, of trusts and monopolies. Medicine too was a business—potentially Big Business. Why not convert the AMA into a giant trust that would dominate the entire healing profession and monopolize medical treatment throughout the U.S.?

He soon realized that the Association, as then set up,

was incapable of assuming such an exalted role. It was constitutionally impotent, little more than a loose federation of state societies over whom it had little say and less control. A radical operation was necessary to transform it into a virile institution capable of fulfilling its destiny.

The editorial pages of the *Journal* began to beat the drums for a reorganization to strengthen the Association and give it exclusive authority to fix medical policy. These editorials attracted the attention of Dr. Joseph N. McCormack of Bowling Green, Ky. Like Simmons, McCormack was more interested in medical politics than in medical practice. Like Simmons, his past was under a cloud. Some years before as Secretary of the Kentucky State Board of Health he'd been arrested in connection with a shortage of $62,000 in his accounts. He didn't even bother to defend himself, it is reported; he merely walked into court and presented a full pardon signed by the Governor.

The two men quickly reached an understanding. McCormack, a close friend of the AMA President-elect, Dr. Charles A. L. Reed, won him over to the project. In 1900, shortly after he took office, Dr. Reed appointed a three-man committee to draw up plans for the reorganization. Two of its members were Simmons and McCormack. An ingeniously calculated plan drafted by this stacked committee was pushed through a convention of politically-innocent physicians the following year.

Only much later, when the smoke cleared, did the members realize that they'd bought a streamlined steamroller made to order for one-man operation—with "Doc" Simmons firmly glued to the driver's seat.

The AMA was reconstructed on three levels: county, state and national. Only at the lowest level did members have a direct voice in their affairs; they elected officers and representatives to a state "legislature." The latter selected delegates to a national "House of Delegates," which in turn picked a nine-man Board of Trustees (each serving 5 years), a President and other officers.

This undemocratic pyramid of power, based on indirect representation and delegation of authority, is the familiar pattern of all authoritarian government. It permits a small, politically-active clique to dominate and control the common herd. This remains today the basic structure of the AMA.

The national officers, elected annually, are merely window-dressing. In an affidavit filed in a U.S. District Court in 1940, AMA President N. V. van Etten confessed:

"My sole office in the AMA is as President. I have no executive or administrative duties in connection with that office, the office being primarily an honorary one, and my chief function as President of the Association being to deliver talks in various parts of the country . . ."

In theory the organization's policies are determined by majority vote of the House of Delegates. Actually this body meets just once a year to rubber-stamp decisions and actions already approved by the Board of Trustees, which functions with little supervision in the interim. The delegates carry policy decisions back to their state societies; these are then turned over to various committees which supervise their implementation and enforcement on the county level.

With the national officers decorative transients, the House of Delegates almost perpetually in recess and the trustees scattered all over the nation attending to their own business, until recently all executive and administrative power fell by default into the hands of an individual who was nominally only a paid employe of the Association: the editor of its *Journal*.

For under the reorganization plan the Journal became the tail that wagged the dog. The national organization collected no dues, its only source of income was the advertising revenue derived from its official organ. It was the editor who okayed all AMA expenditures and signed all AMA checks. Without his approval no official business could be transacted, no policy put in effect, no action whatsoever taken. As usual, he who pays the fiddler calls the tune.

In effect, "Doc" Simmons *was* the AMA.

His first move in his new capacity was a monumental drive to round up and brand every physician in the nation. Dr. McCormack, newly appointed travelling organizer, set out on a journey to prod local societies into activity. By the end of 1903 the Association had tripled in size, total membership was at the 30,000 mark. Two decades later Simmons was able to boast with some justification that he was the "Spokesman for American Medicine"; virtually all the "regular" physicians engaged in private practice in this country were in the AMA. For by now most doctors had learned (as we shall see later) that it was professional suicide *not* to belong to organized medicine.

With the membership campaign well under way, the *Journal* began a rabid crusade against "quacks and charlatans" in the healing profession. Eventually that category came to include all the so-called "irregulars" (drugless physicians, Christian Science practitioners, etc.) as well as "cultists" (osteopaths, chiropractors and—ironically

enough, considering Simmons' own background—homeopathic physicians). In fact any and all unorthodox practitioners.

It turned out to be more of a witch-hunt than a crusade. A private F.B.I., the AMA "Bureau of Investigation,"
was set up to ferret out and "expose" medical heretics.
Poisonous diatribes against them and their methods filled
the *Journal,* slanderous and distorted stories about them
were planted in popular newspapers and magazines. They
were denounced by local medical societies, ostracized by
other members of the profession, harried and harassed by
health inspectors. A high-pressure lobby headed by Dr.
Reed journeyed from state to state whipping up legislation
to limit their professional activities.

The AMA piously proclaimed that its only purpose in
carrying on this ruthless war of extermination was to
protect the public "against medical bandits." But a much
less altruistic incentive is suggested in an intensive legal
study of the Association and its methods published by the
Yale Law Journal (May 1954):

> "(And) although organized medicine's justification for
> limited licensing of the 'cults' is expressed in terms of pro-
> tecting the consumer from unqualified practitioners, there
> may also be present an element of self-protection from eco-
> nomic encroachment."

In plain and simple language its real aim was to eliminate competition and monopolize medical practice.

Laws discriminating against "irregular" medical groups
and restricting their practice were enacted in virtually
every state of the union. Chiropractors were forbidden to
prescribe or administer drugs, puncture the skin or prac-

tice obstetrics. In some states the same limitations applied to osteopaths; in others they were permitted to administer drugs and perform surgery only if they produced proof of "special training." Requirements for the licensing of drugless healers were "discriminatory and inequitable," the Illinois Supreme Court held in 1921, when it ruled the medical practices act of the state "unconstitutional."

However, by this time the medical monopoly was solidly entrenched, and legal machinery to enforce it was in the hands of the monopolists.

AMA standards in medical education, training and practice were adopted by law, and the AMA was empowered to determine whether these standards were met. In most states the law specifies that the head of the Department of Health must be recommended by local medical societies. In at least one state (Alabama) the society itself appoints this public official. In nearly all states local societies are authorized by law to recommend or appoint members of the State Board of Examiners, which has the power to grant or revoke licenses to practice medicine. In Alabama the society's Board of Censors automatically constitutes the official State Board of Medical Examiners.

The state governments, in effect, surrendered all political authority in the field of public health to organized medicine. In the entire history of this country similar power has never been delegated to any other private organization.

It took more than mere talk to persuade state legislatures to turn these powers over to the AMA. Simmons had built up a powerful political machine, and lawmakers in many states quickly discovered that it packed a wicked wallop. Those who incurred disfavor by opposing AMA-sponsored measures (or vice versa) were apt to find themselves out in the cold after election day.

For example, the following excerpt from a report to the AMA refers to the state election in which local doctors spent $50,000 to defeat hostile candidates to the legislature. Its author is Dr. Thomas J. Crowe (whom we'll meet again many times in succeeding chapters), Secretary of the Texas State Board of Medical Examiners:

> "That these campaigns were very effectual we have had ample evidence, since many of those who had opposed public health legislation in the 38th legislature were defeated at the polls; and it was further emphasized when the 39th legislature quickly rendered *hors de combat* the chiropractor biennial bill."

Here is an interesting study in cause and effect, as applied by the AMA, and its influence on legislation affecting the public health!

The quasi-legal status accorded the AMA enabled Simmons to tighten his grip on the profession and complete his strangle-hold on the nation's health by seizing control of two vital outposts of medicine: the medical schools and hospitals.

In 1910, following a report exposing serious inadequacies in medical education, the *Journal* initiated a campaign which put 81 "substandard" schools out of business —and cut in half the number of new doctors graduated annually. Remaining schools were forced to conform to standards set by the AMA Council on Medical Education and submit to regular inspection by AMA inspectors; graduates of institutions not on the Council's approved list were refused licenses to practice medicine by AMA-controlled State Boards.

Thus the AMA acquired the power to dictate what courses shall be given medical students, what they may learn and what their instructors may teach. More than 25 years ago Dr. David L. Edsall, Dean of the Harvard Medical School, sadly told an AMA congress on medical education:

"A little comparison shows that there is less intellectual freedom in the medical course than in almost any other form of professional education in this country."

Even more important from the standpoint of public health, the AMA can dictate the size of classes and thereby control the nation's supply of doctors. During the depression, for example, medical schools all over the country deliberately decreased enrollments "in adherence to the AMA Council's principles." The only principle involved was the Council's concern about a "surplus of doctors."

Today there is an acute shortage of doctors to fulfill the nation's military needs, public health demands and private requirements. Our hospitals need 12,000 internes—there are only 6,000 available. And the shortage steadily grows more alarming. By 1960, according to a U.S. Public Health Bulletin, there will be a deficit of between 17,000 and 45,000 physicians in this country, depending upon the standards we apply.

In no small measure this critical situation is due to the AMA's ability to manipulate the flow of doctors to suit its own economic interest rather than public needs.

Control of the nation's 6,800 registered hospitals passed into AMA hands in much the same fashion: an arbitrary set of standards which have the force of law, periodic inspection by AMA agents, an "accredited" rating that hinged upon carrying out AMA policy.

AMA approval is vital to hospitals. Without it they cannot get internes, because doctors who complete interneship there cannot get licenses in any of the 31 states requiring hospital experience. And AMA doctors will not serve on their staff or send them patients. So even in matters totally unrelated to medical training or treatment, hospitals toe the AMA line.

Such in brief is the powerhouse that Simmons built stage by stage, in accordance with careful design, during his twenty-five year reign over the AMA.

In this relatively short period he transformed an insignificant minority group of 9,000 doctors into a sinister trust that dominated every aspect of American medicine, held a tight grip on the health of the nation and occupied a position of monopoly, authority and influence unequalled by any other professional group in the world.

He turned the AMA *Journal* into one of the most profitable publications in the world, a veritable gold mine of advertising which paid all the expenses of the Association and left a comfortable surplus invested in stocks, bonds and mortgages.

He moved the Association and its official publication out of a single rented room and installed them in their own million-dollar, seven-story steel and concrete citadel that occupied half a block on a main intersection in the heart of Chicago and required a staff of more than 300 employes.

Yet over the years there was growing discontent and disillusion in the ranks of organized medicine. Doctors had surrendered freedom of thought and action, submitted tamely to dictatorship and coercion on the premise that it would improve their economic condition. But they found that little if any of the AMA's rapidly-expanding power, prestige and prosperity sifted down to the level of the average hard-working doctor who made up the bulk of the membership.

In 1922 revolt suddenly broke out in the Illinois Medical Society. An editorial blast headed "THE AMA BECOMES AN AUTOCRACY" appeared in the *Illinois Medical Journal* (Dec. 1922), official publication of the local society. Here is a condensation of its highlights:

"Few of the members of the AMA realize the centralizing changes that have taken place in their organization within the last 25 years. So adroitly and insidiously have these changes been brought about that the majority of the members, dazzled by the material prosperity of the AMA, have entirely overlooked the fact that the Association has been converted from a democratic and self-governed body of professional men into a highly centralized machine with absolute control concentrated in a single individual.

"In the 25 years of expansion of the Association and the *Journal* the anomalous condition has developed whereby the *Journal*, which is the property of the Association, now absolutely controls the Association to which it belongs.

"The editor of the *Journal* has developed into an absolute Dictator of the Association and its affairs through his control of the finances of the Association.

"Measured from a penny-wise standpoint, that the Association has prospered is conceded. But what relation does this temporary financial success bear toward medical ideals, and the betterment of professional conditions?

"In the latter respect, FAILURE IS COMPLETE. That the AMA has done little or nothing for the rank and file of the profession is murmured everywhere and not without justification.

"THE AMA IS NOT A BUSINESS ENTERPRISE.

"Its success is not to be gauged in dollar bills or buildings, but in what it does to benefit its members and retain the confidence and merit the support of physicians.

"In other words, 'What does it profit a man if he gains the whole world and loses his own soul?' What does it profit the AMA to accumulate land, bonds and mortgages with which to erect a whited sepulchre for the genuine interests of the profession it was organized to safeguard?"

Simmons managed to ride out the storm, his supporters gradually reestablished control of the Illinois society. But the handwriting was on the wall.

Less than two years later, when he became involved in an unsavory personal scandal (his wife, also a physician, testified in court that he'd made her a dope addict and tried to railroad her to an insane asylum), the venerable AMA boss was permitted to resign "for reasons of health."

It marked the end of an epoch. Organized medicine as it exists today in this country was largely his creation; for better or worse, it remains his memorial.

The old Dictator was dead, but a new Dictator was born. Simmons' hand-picked successor was his assistant, protégé and faithful disciple: Dr. Morris Fishbein. Since this man plays a prominent role in subsequent chapters of this book, a brief outline of his background and career may be of assistance.

Morris Fishbein was born July 22, 1889 in St. Louis, Mo., the oldest of 8 children. His father, an immigrant peddler, soon moved his rapidly growing family to Indianapolis, where Morris—a rather puny boy—grew up. It was during his last year in high school, his daughter relates, that he decided to become a doctor. A crowd gathered around a man injured in a street brawl, and he joined it. As he tells the story:

"Soon an ambulance drove up, and a little fellow dressed in white with a small black bag jumped out. Immediately the crowd parted for him. I decided to become a doctor."

A very revealing story, and no one who has ever seen him needs a psychiatrist to interpret it. His voracious hunger for power, his insatiable thirst for acceptance and recognition manifest themselves in the man long since he's consumed enough of these to satisfy the appetites of half a dozen ordinary mortals.

At the age of 16 the "little fellow" entered Indiana University Medical School. Badly beaten in a freshman-sophomore roughhouse, he switched to the University of Chicago. After graduation he went to the Rush Medical School where he acquired his M.D. in 1912. New graduates are required to serve a two-year interneship before they are eligible for a medical license in Illinois. Although Fishbein interned for only 5 months before accepting a job as Simmons' assistant at the AMA, he was permitted to take his state board exams.

According to "THE DRUG STORY" by Morris A. Bealle, Fishbein failed to pass his exams but got his license anyway. This is how it was done:

"His boss, George A. Simmons, an advertising quack and abortionist, was a power in Illinois politics at that time. Mr. Fishbein's marks in physical diagnosis, gynecology, etiology and hygiene were left out when his papers were graded. Not so his mark in ANATOMY (the foundation of a medical education) which was 48. By leaving out the low marks in those four subjects the political state board was able to give him a political passing grade and grant him a political medical license."

Fishbein branded this story "a dastardly lie" during his trial for slander and libel (see Chapter 15); he declared his grade in anatomy was 65. He finally was forced to admit that 65 wasn't a passing score, either.

Be that as it may, he never practiced medicine a day in his life. He wasn't interested in treating patients. With cold, unerring instinct he headed straight for the real source of power, prestige and cash in the field of medicine: the AMA. He worked hard, made himself indispensable, understudied his boss for 11 years and bided his time. When the bell tolled for the old man, his 35-year-old understudy was well prepared to take over the job editing the AMA *Journal* without a hitch or break in rhythm.

And he quickly demonstrated that he was a worthy heir to the mantle of authority that went by precedent with his new job.

Up to this time the AMA had no public relations or press program. Fishbein immediately stepped into the limelight as supersalesman for the AMA way of life to the American people. He created a smooth, well-oiled publicity machine that ground out an unending stream of press releases, "canned" speeches and debates on political as well as medical subjects, newspaper columns, magazine articles and radio broadcasts. He blanketed the country with AMA propaganda, utilizing every means of public communication to extol and defend organized medicine and to defame its enemies.

The witch-hunt against unorthodox medicine was accelerated and became more venomous than ever. To Fishbein anyone in the healing profession outside the AMA was "scum of the earth," and he pursued heretics with a zeal reminiscent of the Spanish Inquisition. He maintained a card index of 300,000 "medical fakers"—including many reputable doctors who had resigned or been ousted from the AMA. No accusation, however vile, was too vicious to be hurled against them; no manufactured "evidence," however fake, too putrid a device to destroy them.

A Texas District Court characterized the charges he made against the Hoxsey treatment as "untruthful, slanderous and libelous" (see Chapter 15). And he made similar wild charges against other opponents in various disputes. For example:

In 1932 he attacked a report by the Committee on the Costs of Medical Care as *socialism and communism, inciting to revolution.* The "subversive" who headed that committee happened to be Dr. Ray Lyman Wilbur, President of Stanford University, former U.S. Secretary of the Interior—and past president of the AMA itself!

In 1948, on his return from England, he published and broadcast over the air a highly unfavorable report on government health insurance as he'd seen it in practice there. The British Medical Association promptly made public a letter branding his report a lie and a "libel."

The AMA campaign against group health plans (allegedly because they violated the principles of "free enterprise") demonstrated that freedom of opinion and action within the AMA membership was nil. Doctors who supported or participated professionally in such plans were expelled by their local societies and, by AMA decree, were denied privileges in all "approved" hospitals.

Thus in Milwaukee a hospital superintendent who kept several expelled doctors on his staff was notified that the institution would be removed from the "approved interne list" if he didn't get rid of them. He immediately did so.

In Washington, D.C., a hospital refused to admit the patient of an expelled doctor for an emergency operation because AMA members threatened to move their patients out of the hospital.

In the state of Washington a hospital denied an expelled doctor the use of its facilities, forcing him to take his seriously ill patient through a snow storm to a distant hospital.

Such practices caused the U.S. Supreme Court in 1940 to find the AMA guilty of violating the anti-trust laws, and formally enjoin it from continuing the violation. It didn't stay enjoined. More than 10 years later (1952) a similar decision by the Washington State Supreme Court demonstrated that local medical societies were still engaged in the same monopoly practice.

His official position brought Fishbein great prestige which he exploited and commercialized to the hilt. He allegedly wrote 30,000 words a week under his own byline (in which he invariably identified himself as "Editor of the AMA *Journal*") for publication in popular newspapers and magazines, and he collected the usual author's fees (or better). Although he never practiced medicine or treated a patient, he had no hesitation in setting himself up as an authority on all kinds of human illness and treatments. His daily column of medical advice, syndicated in newspapers all over the country, always contained a box which suggested:

"Save Dr. Fishbein's articles from day to day and paste them in a scrap book. In a short time you will find you have acquired an invaluable modern home medical guide with reliable information on every health question."

The California Medical Society protested. It said Fishbein's column not only commercialized the AMA, but was *full of medical inaccuracies and misstatements!*

A prolific hack writer, he authored 18 popular books on subjects ranging from soap to syphilis, from medical writing to sex advice (four of them in one year); he co-authored two more, and edited six others. Newspaper ads for his *Modern Home Medical Adviser* were so extravagantly phrased that they caused an uproar in the New York Medical Society; charges of "false and misleading advertising" were filed with the Federal Trade Commission; Sen. Pepper denounced the whole exhibition as "charlatanism."

This was the final blow—the man who called others a quack himself accused of quackery! He meekly conceded: *"It (the advertising) was most unfortunate. I told the publisher to change it at once."* Unfortunate was scarcely the word for it, his critics snorted; it was disgraceful! Especially since any other doctor whose name even appeared in the lay press was subject to charges of "self-advertising."

His job as newspaper columnist for various syndicates, medical editor of *Good Housekeeping* and "adviser" to numerous other popular magazines put Fishbein in close touch with science writers and enabled him to exert considerable influence on their writings. On Oct. 30, 1937, the AMA Board of Trustees played host to the National Association of Science Writers at a special conference allegedly to discuss ways and means *"to keep the public informed of progress in medical science."* The aim, of course, was exactly the opposite. Soon thereafter the writers' association adopted as part of its "code of ethics" the following principle:

"Science writers are incapable of judging the facts of phenomena involved in medical and scientific discovery. Therefore they only report 'discoveries' approved by medical authorities, or those presented before a body of scientific peers."

This voluntary censorship of medical news *not* approved by "medical authorities" (i.e. the AMA) was accepted by the leading news services. For example, in 1940 the United Press sent out a bulletin to its various bureaus all over the country which ordered, in part:

"Under no circumstances put any story on the leased wire about a remedy. If the bureau manager is convinced that the story has merit, he should overhead it to New York for investigation and consideration there."

The only "investigation" such a story received was a query to the AMA; if the latter disapproved, the story never appeared.

The conspiracy to censor vital medical news was exposed August, 1954, in testimony before the House Committee on Veterans' Affairs. Arthur J. Connell, National Commander of the American Legion, told Congress that

". . . a contract exists between the State medical associations and the newspapers which makes it virtually impossible for the veterans' side of medical questions to reach the reading public."

He read the contract into the record. It stipulated that *"on all matters of health and medical news"* no publication or radio broadcast would be made until *"authentic information"* is obtained from *"qualified sources"* named in the agreement. These "qualified sources," of course, are AMA officials. To illustrate how this agreement works, Connell cited an editorial attacking medical aid to war veterans, published by the Denver *Post*. He said this editorial, on investigation, proved to be written by an official of the Colorado State Medical Society.

Although most concerned about suppression and distortion of news affecting veterans, Connell pointed out that all other medical news not approved by the AMA is handled in the same manner, and has no way of reaching the public.

No wonder the Hoxsey treatment, and other unorthodox methods, never get a favorable hearing in our "free" but medically-censored press.

A very busy man by any standards, Fishbein still found time to occupy professorial posts as lecturer at the University of Chicago Medical School and the University of Illinois College of Medicine. The "little fellow" who by his own admission couldn't make a passing grade in anatomy in his state board exams had come a long way indeed!

And it had paid off—handsomely. It is estimated that his income from extra-curricular duties (including book royalties) at least tripled the pay he received from the AMA ($24,000 per year). That, as the man says, ain't hay.

Fishbein, like his predecessor, ruled the AMA for 25 years. And like Simmons during that time he acquired many critics and enemies within the organization. As far back as 1938 the New Jersey Medical Society passed a resolution urging that he be ordered to confine his writings to the *Journal.* It and subsequent anti-Fishbein resolutions introduced by other state societies went down before the steamroller at AMA conventions. Few even reached the floor for a vote.

The culminating battle of his career—and the one that directly led to his downfall—was the titanic struggle against government health insurance. The AMA had fought the spectre of government intervention in the field of medical practice—which would have signed the death warrant of its monopoly—for more than 20 years. In 1944 it had set up a permanent lobby in Washington to keep Congress in line, and by strenuous efforts this lobby had managed to keep various health insurance bills bottled up in committee. But popular demand for government action to provide medical care for those who couldn't afford it kept right on growing.

Fishbein threw all his resources and boundless energy into the struggle—thundering editorials in the *Journal*, alarming articles in newspapers and magazines, blustering speeches before civic groups and slippery debates over the radio. He galloped around the country with the cry that the Bolsheviks were coming. His best efforts to drag the red herring across the trail of free discussion (he called health insurance "Communism" in 1929, "Nazism" in 1939 and "Communism" again in 1949) by this time had taken on the aspect of low comedy routine.

And in slug-fests over the air with prominent advocates of the bill, he was hopelessly out-classed. They tripped him up on contrary statements and statistics, nailed him with misrepresentation of fact and outright lies, made him (and the AMA) sound ridiculous to radio audiences.

Slowly the conviction grew in conservative administrative circles of the AMA that the egocentric little man was a liability to their cause. The only way to kill government health insurance for good was to rally public opinion against it. The public considered Fishbein "the symbol of old reactionary leadership," and wouldn't go along with him. The Board of Trustees had to act.

At the convention in June, 1949, he was permitted to retire for the usual "reasons of health"—at the ripe old age of 60. Adding insult to injury, the announcement specified that he was not to speak, write or be interviewed "on controversial subjects." As one witty writer put it (*Harper's*, Nov. 1949):

> "Last June the AMA withdrew its seal of approval from Morris Fishbein. Then, just so there would be no misunderstanding, it beat his head in, cut his heart out and kicked him into the street. 'If the atmosphere becomes unpleasant,' said the Voice of American Medicine, picking himself up and straightening his necktie, 'I'll quit in five minutes.'"

With that out of the way, the AMA proceeded with its campaign to kill the health bill. It already had collected a $3½ million war chest by slapping a tax of $25 on each of its 140,000 members. (Those who refused to pay were threatened with expulsion.) Its Washington office was greatly expanded, a small army of lobbyists descended on Congress.

A "National Educational Campaign" directed by a firm of high-pressure public relations experts was launched to arouse the public to the evils of "socialized medicine," and a special staff of 37 employes was set up in Chicago to plan and coordinate the drive.

Soon nearly every doctor in the land displayed Campaign posters, distributed Campaign literature in his waiting room, mailed Campaign leaflets to patients with their monthly bills. Doctors' wives were urged to *"tuck pamphlets into all personal correspondence—even invitations to dinner parties."* Physicians of Congressmen personally contacted them and urged them to vote against the bill. (Rep. John Dinglel of Michigan charged that this was *"taking advantage of a special confidential relationship to lobby."*)

Less than a year later Campaign headquarters proudly announced that propaganda literature had been distributed to over 100 million people at a cost of about a million dollars!

County and state medical societies organized public meetings for which they supplied speakers and text. They solicited local editorial support, purchased space in newspapers and time on the radio. They induced prominent civic and business organizations to pass resolutions against "socialized medicine" and showered Congress with copies of these resolutions.

By the end of the year a total of 1,829 separate organizations—ranging in size from a handful to 5 million members—had endorsed the AMA crusade.

Members of Congress were deluged with letters, telegrams and telephone calls from constituents. They were button-holed, badgered and bedevilled by lobbyists. Few of them could stand up under such pressure; one by one they threw in the sponge. Before the session closed the bill's proponents sadly admitted that they couldn't muster enough votes to get it passed, and gave up the unequal struggle.

But the AMA wasn't through with them yet. The Congressional elections of 1950 were coming up, and Congress was going to learn the hard way that it must play ball with organized medicine—or else.

Now the Association and its component societies are banned by their charter as non-profit corporations from engaging in political activities. A few months before the elections the AMA gave every member a copy of a memorandum prepared by a Chicago legal firm, informing them that there was nothing in the law to prevent doctors as individuals from endorsing or working for any candidate. The inference was plain.

All over the nation they organized "Healing Arts," "Medical Dental" and similar committees. They worked day and night to shelve candidates who'd supported health insurance; they distributed campaign literature, advertised in local newspapers, addressed election rallies. In Florida, where they opposed Sen. Claude Pepper's renomination, hospital patients found cards on their breakfast trays with the pregnant message: "This is the season for canning Pepper!"

During the week of October 8th the AMA put on a whirlwind advertising campaign that cost $1,100,000. Ostensibly directed against compulsory health insurance, it was timed strategically to influence Congressional elections. AMA copy attacking "socialized medicine" and its advocates appeared in more than 10,000 daily and weekly newspapers throughout the country, in 35 magazines, was broadcast over 1,600 radio stations. An additional $2 million in tie-in advertising was subscribed by banks, insurance and utility companies, medical supply houses and pharmaceutical firms.

When the final election results were in, the AMA had

won a resounding victory. Sen. Pepper in Florida, Sen. Graham in North Carolina, Rep. Biemiller in Wisconsin and a host of other Federal health insurance advocates in many states had been thoroughly trounced.

The AMA's president called the elections *"very reassuring"* and predicted that *"any compulsory health insurance bill in Congress today would go down to defeat by at least a 2 to 1 vote."* Actually this was an understatement. When such a bill was introduced the following year, it never got out of committee.

Congress had learned its lesson. It knew that the AMA is bad medicine when it's crossed.

If anyone thought for a moment that dropping its reactionary pilot meant that the AMA was changing course, he was due for a rude awakening. The monopolistic techniques of the Association, originated by Simmons and perfected by Fishbein, have not changed. The AMA still dominates medical schools and hospitals, it still fights unorthodox practitioners tooth and nail, it still maintains a powerful lobby to fight social reform and government intervention in matters of public health.

And it is still an oligarchy dominated by a small clique of medico-politicians. The average honest, hard-working doctor still has little or no voice in its affairs.

According to a recent survey, over 90 percent of the Association's officers are prosperous specialists, and the vast majority of those who serve long terms in the House of Delegates come from urban areas. Enjoying incomes much higher than that of the average practitioner, they are able to devote more time to medical politics. They make up the hierarchy of the AMA, they are the policy makers. And the policies they adopt further their own interests, rather than the interests of the average doctor (let alone the interests of the public).

Short of revolution, the faction in control of the AMA cannot be removed from office. It is practically self-perpetuating.

AMA election procedures give the officers in power a decisive influence in naming their successors. At each level—county, state and national—the President appoints a nominating committee which draws up an official slate of officers and delegates. Opposition slates are seldom permitted, electioneering and soliciting votes for office is strictly forbidden. Thus the same names appear on the ballot year after year. And officers who prove "reliable" are promoted from county, to state, to national position as they acquire seniority.

Doctors who oppose official policy find no way to effectuate their views within the rigid framework of the organization. The AMA *Journal* consistently refuses to print opposition discussion; and any attempt to obtain a hearing in lay periodicals is punished by ouster from the ranks of organized medicine.

Theoretically, dissidents can press their viewpoints at the local level. If they can win over a majority there, it can be carried to the state level, and then to the national. In practice, this is a farce. Even at local levels opposition is squelched before it can get started. As one local society official bluntly told an AMA gathering:

"You would be surprised how little democracy there is in most county societies."

The victims of the AMA are not alone the general public and unorthodox practitioners; in the first instance they are to be found in the rank and file membership of the organization. America's doctors have abjectly surrendered freedom of opinion and professional action. They dare not voice scientific theories or espouse methods which are not approved by the AMA. To do so means economic suicide.

And this was the outfit I antagonized in 1924, when I refused to let Dr. Harris and his AMA associates take over the Hoxsey treatment. That was the beginning of a 35-year war, which still continues today.

CHAPTER NINE

Struggle for Survival

THE DOOR to acceptance and an honorable career, only yesterday wide ajar, had been slammed rudely in my face. Disappointed but grimly determined that nothing and no one on God's green earth would prevent me from curing cancer, I prepared to return to Taylorville and proceed with our original plan to build a bigger and better clinic there.

At this point Lucius Everhard, the insurance broker who provided our original contact with Dr. Harris, stepped in and urged us to transfer our activities to Chicago. Here, in what many consider the "medical capital of the world," the AMA maintains national headquarters; here our fight for medical recognition could be waged more effectively. Everhard had discussed the situation with wealthy friends, and they were willing to finance a research institute and clinic for the Hoxsey method.

We decided to accept the offer. A common law trust was set up with Everhard as chairman of the board of trustees and one of his friends, R. M. Wilbur, as business manager. Dr. Miller was retained as medical director, and I nominally as "technical advisor." We wound up our affairs in Taylorville as quickly as possible and on October 1, 1924, opened offices in the Mallers Building, within half a mile of the national stronghold of organized medicine on North Dearborn Street.

It took me just one month to discover that Everhard and his cohorts had only one interest in my cancer treatment: to convert it into a get-rich-quick racket. Our new business manager set fees ranging from $500 to $1,000 per case. Even worse, contrary to our original agreement he was turning away all charity patients, refusing our treatment to unfortunates who couldn't afford to pay cash on the barrel-head.

In a stormy session with Everhard and Wilbur I accused them of exploiting human suffering and misery for personal gain and handed them an ultimatum.

"This isn't a fly-by-night quack treatment," I told them, "it's a legitimate cure for cancer. And I intend to make it available to everyone, regardless of how much or how little money they have. Cancer makes no distinction between poor and rich; poor people suffer from it just as much as rich people, their lives are just as important to them and their families, they deserve the same chance to get effective treatment. Either they get it here or I'll get out and see that they get it elsewhere."

Everhard smiled cynically. "Those are mighty fine sentiments, my friend, but they won't buy you any groceries. Don't be a sucker. Your treatment's a gold mine. Leave the business details to us and we'll make you a millionaire in spite of yourself!"

"I don't want any part of that kind of money!" I retorted angrily and walked out.

To my surprise and dismay Dr. Miller, instead of sharing my indignation, attempted to placate me. "You can't fight the world single-handed, Harry. We've got to be practical. It takes money to battle the AMA. These people are your friends, they'll help you put over your treatment."

"God save me from such friends," I quoted bitterly, "I'll take care of my enemies myself."

I immediately severed my connection with this rich man's clinic and cut off its supply of medicine. Thoroughly disgusted and disillusioned with Chicago, evidently just another small-town boy ripe for plucking by big-city slickers, I packed my bags and went home.

Taylorville tendered its prodigal son an enthusiastic welcome. The Chamber of Commerce passed a resolution expressing confidence in Harry Hoxsey and his method of treating cancer. Local businessmen volunteered enough money to set up a new cancer clinic and hospital; the Moose Lodge gave me a long-term lease on its home with an option for eventual purchase.

Early in 1925 the remodelled and redecorated building was ready, and the Hoxide Institute opened its doors. Its medical director was Dr. Wilbur Washburn, a reputable and able local physician. Our maximum fee was fixed at $300 and no one was turned away because he couldn't afford to pay.

The local Chamber of Commerce launched a vigorous campaign to make Taylorville the cancer capital of America. A committee headed by H. C. Moxley collected affidavits from 30 former Hoxsey patients and reprinted them in a booklet which it sent out by the thousands to other Chambers of Commerce throughout the country. In addition it sponsored a series of advertisements in mid-western newspapers urging cancer victims everywhere to communicate with its Secretary for authoritative information about treatment "under strictly ethical medical supervision, painlessly, without operation and with permanent results."

As a result patients began to come in from all parts of the United States and Canada.

Then the AMA struck its first blow.

That summer—a few months after the opening of our new clinic—a stranger appeared in Taylorville and interviewed a number of the town's leading citizens, making inquiries about me, my family and our treatment. He identified himself as an agent of the AMA Bureau of Investigation. As nearly everyone he talked with had been treated for cancer by me or my father, or had relatives or friends who owed their lives to the Hoxsey treatment, he heard nothing but praise and confidence in our ability to cure cancer.

Informed of his activities, I sent word to him that he was welcome to visit our clinic, get the personal information he sought first-hand, question patients, see the work we were doing and judge for himself the results. He never showed up, nor even acknowledged my invitation. A few days later I learned that he'd skulked out of town as stealthily as he had come in.

Months passed and the year ended without any further sign of interest by the AMA, so I assumed its investigator had been unable to dig up anything detrimental to me or my treatment.

Suddenly on Jan. 2, 1926, the official *Journal* of the AMA came out with a three-page blast at the Hoxide Institute. Ostensibly an official report by the Association's Bureau of Investigation, it was in fact a scurrilous, slanderous smear attack upon me, my father, the Hoxsey treatment and everyone at any time associated with us.

Among the numerous distortions, half-truths and outright lies were the following:

That my father was a *"quack"* who'd dabbled in veterinary medicine, *"faith healing and cancer curing";* that he'd been arrested on a charge of blackmailing a local dentist but *"somehow escaped punishment";* that he himself had died of cancer!

That the Hoxsey treatment *"ate into the blood vessels"* and some of our patients *"bled to death";* that in at least two unspecified cases it destroyed tissue and bone and caused death!

That patients we proclaimed as cured never had cancer; they were simply afflicted with *"non-malignant or superficial growths!"*

Dumbfounded by this cowardly attempt at character assassination, more suited to a yellow scandal sheet than an allegedly scientific journal, I immediately sat down and addressed a furious reply to Dr. Morris Fishbein, editor of the AMA *Journal.*

I pointed out that my father indeed had once been falsely accused of attempted blackmail. However there were court records to prove that he was innocent and had been exonerated of the charge. The claim that he'd died of cancer was equally false; his death certificate, on file at the State Capital, would show that he'd died of erysipelas.

I defied Dr. Fishbein to name even one specific case in which my treatment ate into blood vessels and caused death by hemorrhage. I demanded that he make public the names and medical records of the two anonymous patients who allegedly died as the result of destruction of tissue and bone by our treatment.

As for the charge that the people we cured never really had cancer, I dared Dr. Fishbein to publish the medical records in the Mannix case, certified as a true cancer by none other than a prominent official of the AMA. And I challenged him to publish the records of scores of other cases diagnosed as cancer by AMA doctors and successfully treated by the Hoxsey method.

Finally I invited the AMA to send a group of outstanding cancer experts to inspect our files, examine our patients, observe our treatment and make a fair and unbiased estimate of the results we obtained. The only conditions attached were that their conclusions be based on facts, naming names and citing chapter and verse in each case; and that their report—either for or against me—be published in full in the AMA *Journal*. Then the whole medical profession could judge whether our treatment was a fake or a real cure for cancer.

Dr. Fishbein never replied to my letter. Nor did he ever publish any of the indicated medical records. Instead of a fair and impartial investigation, the AMA opened a well-oiled campaign to discredit me and put the Hoxide Institute out of business.

Reprints of the medical journal smear were sent to every member of the Taylorville Chamber of Commerce, accompanied by a letter from the County Medical Society urging local businessmen to repudiate their endorsement and withdraw their support from our clinic. Shortly thereafter a high-pressured AMA hatchetman from Chicago appeared at a meeting of the Chamber and delivered a harangue in which he said, among other things, that each of its members would be morally and legally responsible for the death of our patients if the literature didn't stop.

"He didn't get very far," my friend Fred Baugh, secretary of the organization, reported with a grin. "We don't scare easy. I stood up and told how Hoxsey cured me of cancer. Then Fred Auchenbach told what you'd done for him, how at least a dozen others in this town would be dead and gone now if it wasn't for the Hoxsey treatment. Then old man Larkin rared back and spoke his piece, told that fellow that the whole county knew the stuff they printed about your daddy was a pack of lies, they could see for themselves you're curing cancer. When we called for a show of hands on the question, by gum there wasn't a single one raised against you!"

As long as the Chamber of Commerce stood by me, the AMA knew it would have a tough time closing down my clinic. Seeking ways and means of leaping that hurdle, its agents came up with an ingenious plan. And they found a willing tool to help them put it over: Harvey Gallagher, cashier of the Colgrave State Bank in Taylorville.

At a business meeting a few weeks later Gallagher introduced a stranger from Chicago allegedly interested in "bringing up to date" all business organizations in the state. The stranger said that a new "Association of Commerce" had been formed to take over the functions of local Chambers of Commerce and integrate their activities. The bank cashier introduced a resolution that the Taylorville Chamber be dissolved, its members receive a refund of their original initiation fee ($25) and affiliate themselves with the new Association. This resolution was passed, and Gallagher was elected secretary of the local branch.

Then the joker in the deck appeared.

Among the by-laws of the "Association" was one prohibiting member groups from endorsing any private institution. Gallagher immediately stopped the mailing of literature in favor of the Hoxide Institute; when letters requesting information came in, he dictated evasive replies. The real purpose of the reorganization now clear, my friends protested vigorously but in vain. Many members—including Baugh and Auchenbach—resigned in disgust. But it was too late. The AMA had achieved its purpose, it had destroyed official support of the Hoxsey treatment.

(Significantly enough, a few years later Harvey Gallagher was convicted of absconding with funds deposited at his bank, and sent to the penitentiary. After his release he admitted to me that the entire maneuver with the Chamber or Commerce had been directed by organized medicine.)

But the medical association soon discovered that it had won a hollow victory. Business at the clinic was affected only slightly, for nobody could stop patients who took our treatment from spreading the word that we actually cured cancer. Within a few months we were operating at full capacity again.

One hot day in July a stranger came into the clinic and handed me his card. It read: *"Emil Johnstone, Carlinville, Ill., Investigator, State Medical Board."* He asked to see our medical licenses and I showed him Dr. Washburn's hanging on the wall. Then he asked for mine. I looked him squarely in the eye.

"I have none, except the license of any American citizen to work at his trade. I'm a technician, I work under the supervision of Dr. Washburn."

"That's a damned lie, Hoxsey, and you know it!" he burst out. "You're the whole works here, you're practicing medicine without a license and we're going to close you up!"

"Just try and do it!" I challenged.

He turned on his heel and stalked out.

That night I drove to Springfield to attend a movie. As I came out of the theatre I heard a newsboy shouting the headlines: "FAKE CANCER CLINIC RAIDED!" Another boy was yelling "DOWNSTATE MURDER MILL RAIDED!" Snatching up copies of the papers, I read that the Sheriff's office had closed the Hoxide Institute, that a warrant was out for my arrest. One of the papers even had me already in jail. All of them carried lurid tales about patients who died "as the result" of our treatment. (Of course, some of our patients died; we never pretended we could cure them all.) But there was no mention of the fact that practically all our cases previously had been declared incurable by their own doctors—nor of the many patients we had cured.

Speeding back to Taylorville, I stopped at our clinic. The sleepy attendant who answered my ring was surprised when I showed him the headlines. He said there had been no raid, as I could see our hospital was still open and operating normally.

I got the Sheriff, Andy Fletcher, on the phone. He too was surprised. "It's news to me," he declared. "There's no warrant here for your arrest."

The following morning I called the editors of the newspapers, informed them that no action had been taken against me or my clinic and demanded an explanation. They informed me they had it on "reliable authority" that the Illinois Medical Board had sworn out a warrant for my arrest and had closed the clinic. I told them that unless they printed a retraction I would sue for libel.

Two nights later a lawyer from Springfield walked into the Sheriff's office and handed Deputy Sheriff Ben Kerns a warrant for my arrest on the charge of practicing medicine without a license. Ben read it very carefully, aimed a stream of tobacco juice at the brass cuspidor three feet away, contemptuously tossed the document down on the desk.

"That boy's been treating me for cancer," he announced. "If you think I'm going to serve a warrant on a fellow who's saving my life, you've got another think coming!"

Taken aback, the lawyer insisted on talking to the Sheriff. Ben jerked his head toward the phone. "Help yourself, Mister," he snapped, and turned his back.

Later that evening Sheriff Fletcher phoned me at home to inform me that there was a warrant out for my arrest. "I told that lawyer I had a touch of lumbago and couldn't get around to the office 'til morning," he said. "Maybe not before noon. Better call your lawyer. And get in touch with Fred Auchenbach or 'Tip' Larkin; you'll need about $500 bond money. Call me after you've got it."

I thanked him, went to·work on the telephone. Bright and early the next morning, accompanied by my lawyer, I walked into the Sheriff's office, handed over a signed and sealed bail bond for $500 and walked out again.

The case went to the Grand Jury about a week later. Two of the twelve members of that jury had taken the Hoxsey treatment and been cured of cancer; each of the others had relatives or friends who'd taken the treatment. They heard the evidence, promptly handed down their verdict:

"It's not against the law to save people's lives. Indictment not warranted."

Within two months no fewer than seven warrants against me were sworn out on the same charge. Yet I never spent a day in jail, not a single one of these cases ever reached trial. And the clinic continued to operate as usual. Then the plague of warrants abruptly abated, winter came and went without any further show of hostilities.

The next—and most damaging—blow came from a totally unexpected quarter.

CHAPTER TEN

Family Squabble

One fine morning in the Spring of 1927 while on my way to the clinic I saw the short, squat figure of Deputy Sheriff Ben Kerns deliberately easing his ponderous bulk down the street just ahead. As I caught up he glanced around warily, shifted the ever-present cud to the other side of his mouth and said casually:

"I'm on my way to serve you with a court order tying up everything you got—prop'ty, cash, the whole caboodle. But I ain't seen you, un'erstand? Get busy, I'll be down by the clinic again in a couple of hours and my eyesight might improve some."

"What's the charge, Ben?"

"Trover." He spat noisily.

"Never heard of it. What's that?"

He shrugged. "Dunno, but it sounds serious. Get your lawyer. And put your bank account and such-like out of sight so it can't be attached." He winked and walked away.

I made a bee-line for the Taylorville National Bank, which handled my account. As I was about to enter the door a young fellow I knew quite well, Guy Jennings, stopped me.

"Harry," he said apologetically, extending a bulky document, "I got something for you. It came in the mail today. A lawyer in Springfield by the name of Templeman sent it to me to serve on you." I remembered that Guy occasionally made a few dollars extra as a process server.

"What is it?"

"Summons and complaint. Hell, Harry, I hate to do this to you. Say the word and I'll let on I can't find you."

"Never mind. Might as well get it over with." I took the papers and glanced at them.

The word *"trover"* met my eye. It still didn't mean a thing to me. But when I found the names of the plaintiffs I went cold with shock. They were Mrs. Mattie Voyles and Mrs. Belle Boyer of Springfield; James R. Hoxsey, Mrs. George (Viola) Trojack and Mrs. Walter (Nora) McClughan, of Taylorville; and Mrs. Nellie Vorbeck of Plymouth, Michigan.

All my brothers and sisters—every one of them, except William. They were suing me for $500,000, the alleged value of their share of my father's estate which I, according to this complaint, had *"illegally appropriated."* But that estate was settled in 1920, and consisted of little more than debts!

Then the answer came to me: the formulas Dad had entrusted to my keeping!

I forgot all about the bank and Ben Kerns waiting for me at the clinic with a writ of attachment, was off like a shot for Nora's house. My favorite sister, who had taken me into her house when Mother died. Never a whisper of disagreement between us. Yet she'd signed this, never told me about it!

Bursting in through the front door, I found her in the tiny parlor where a big portrait of our father hung on the wall. I slapped the paper down on the table before her. "Did you sign that?"

Her face went white, she clasped her hands to keep them from trembling. "Brother," she stammered, "I had to. They came here and kept after me—all three of them. . . ."

"Who?" I demanded.

"A lawyer from Springfield, a Mr. Templeman. And two other lawyers from Chicago, a Mr. Blake and a Mr. Kirk. They said if I didn't sign I'd be a party to the suit anyway, and we'd lose our home and new car and everything we own, and Walter would lose his job. . . ."

"And you fell for that?"

Nora was miserable. "I didn't know what to do," she pleaded. "Mattie called from Springfield and said it was the best thing for everybody concerned, including yourself. Instead of wearing yourself out fighting the doctors' league, you'd get $50,000 along with the rest of us . . ."

I thought she'd suddenly gone mad. "Wait a minute now. What do you mean, $50,000?"

She nodded eagerly. "Sure, they told us as soon as the suit was settled and we won shares in the cancer formulas they'd buy us out, give us each $50,000 for our interest."

"Who'd buy you out?"

"They said a group of prominent doctors in Chicago was interested in the treatment. . . ."

The light suddenly dawned on me. So that was the explanation for the acute interest of the two lawyers from Chicago in this matter. Failing in their attempt to negotiate and equally unsuccessful in their efforts to pressure me out, the medical hierarchy had connived this legal gimmick for the sole purpose of getting their hands on the Hoxsey treatment so they could exploit it and enrich themselves at the expense of humanity.

Torn between anger and sorrow, I listened intently as Nora told me the whole story.

It began when our sister Mattie (Mrs. Voyles) who lived in Springfield consulted an attorney named Templeman about a divorce. The lawyer was quite unenthusiastic when she told him that she couldn't afford the fee he set. But when he learned that her maiden name was Hoxsey, and that she was a sister of *"that fellow in Taylorville who runs a cancer cure,"* he suddenly displayed keen interest. Questioning her closely, he drew from her the full story of the origin of the Hoxsey treatment.

A few days later he called her in and introduced her to Blake and Kirk, the Chicago lawyers. They told her that she and the rest of the family had a legal right to a share in the Hoxsey treatment because it was part of our father's estate. The old family formulas were worth a lot of money; in fact they knew a group of doctors who were willing to pay each heir $50,000 for his share. Moreover, out of the goodness of their hearts they'd foot all the expenses of a legal suit to compel me to give each member of the family his "rightful share."

Depressed by personal unhappiness and dazzled by this sudden prospect of wealth, Mattie signed the complaint. Then the three lawyers went to work on the rest of the family with cajolery, promises and threats until they too signed. All except Will, who declared flatly he wouldn't have any part in the proceedings and stubbornly refused to be budged.

"But you all know that Dad gave me the formulas," I cried indignantly. "Not one of you ever showed the slightest interest in the cancer treatment while he was still alive. And when he died, all you cared about was the money left after the debts were paid. You wouldn't have known what to do with the formulas if you had them, they'd be lost and forgotten by now except for all the sweat and struggle I've put in!"

Nora bowed her head, sighed wearily. "Yes, we all know that, and we told the lawyers so. But they insist the law says different, that these formulas are family property and Dad had no right to give them away."

"We'll see about that!" I asserted grimly, getting to my feet.

Tears in her eyes, she put her hand timidly on my arm. "Harry, why keep butting your head against a stone wall? You can't lick the whole world. Let them have the formulas. I don't want the money, you can have my share, I'm sure the rest of the family feel the same way. All we want is peace, to be let alone."

"Nora," I said quietly, trying hard to suppress my anger, "you know what I promised Dad just before he died. I wouldn't break that promise for fifty million dollars. No, not for all the money in the world. So it's peace you all want? And you want it so bad you'll lie for it, and let a bunch of thieving rascals steal our birthright? Not me. I'm going to fight for my rights!"

I left, made my way to the bank and telephoned my lawyer, John Hogan. He came right over, and we went into Fred Auchenbach's office for a conference.

I was really on the spot this time, Hogan told me after reading the complaint. Bond covering the entire amount demanded in the action ($500,000) had to be raised immediately, or all my assets—personal and business— would be attached pending trial. The bond could be cash, or real estate. The latter was acceptable at half its appraised value. In other words a million dollars worth of real estate must be put up as security.

I looked at the banker. He was one of the people who'd promised to stand back of me if I ever got into trouble because I had treated him for cancer.

"That's a lot of money, Harry. I don't see how you can raise it. Not in Taylorville. Take my house. It's worth $40,000, but for tax purposes it's appraised at only $18,-000. I have a $10,000 mortgage on it, so that leaves only $8,000 clear. But the courts'll allow only $4,000 on it as bond, just a drop in the bucket considering what you need. The same goes for property owned by 'Tip' Larkin, old man McVicker and your other friends. We said we'd back you to the limit, and we will. But they've boosted the ante beyond our reach."

I stared glumly at my shoes. No mistaking it, I was in for trouble. And my friends couldn't help me; I'd have to fight it out alone.

The phone rang. It was my wife (I'd been married a couple of months before). She said three men were at our house with a court writ authorizing them to list every stick of furniture, household goods and personal possessions. Hogan nodded: let them do it. I repeated this to my wife, told her not to worry, I'd explain when I got home.

Fred Auchenbach said: "Let's get busy now. Assign your bank account to me. Assign all your accounts receivable, I'll collect them and hold them in your name.

When you need money don't draw a check, come to me."

Signing the necessary papers I remarked, with a wry smile: "The way them doctors in Chicago are awheelin' and adealin' to get the formulas from me, you'd never guess my treatment kills instead of cures, like the medical journal says it does. Looks like they don't believe their own propaganda!"

"I'm walking proof it's a lie," the banker declared, tapping his left breast where the cancer had been removed by my treatment.

My car was parked across the street from the bank. As I started to get in, Ben Kerns lumbered over.

"All set now?" he yawned.

"Guess so."

"Now 'bout that automobile? That in your name?"

I nodded.

"Get rid of it, ye derned fool. I'm goin' down to the depot. See you in a little while."

I telephoned Clair Nightingale at the Star Motor Company in Decatur, 20 miles away, where I'd bought the car, and explained the circumstances. He told me to hold everything, he'd be right over with a repossess. Within half an hour he arrived at the clinic, thrust a notarized paper at me. I signed on the dotted line.

A few minutes later Ben Kerns ambled in. "Mr. Hoxsey," he said in his best official manner, "I got a possess order for your automobile."

"Just a minute, Sheriff," the auto dealer intervened, waving the paper I'd just signed. "That there car don't belong to Hoxsey, it's mine. He couldn't keep up the payments and I had to replevin it."

"Wal, now, that's too bad," the Deputy sighed. "Ef

you don't own a car, Mr. Hoxsey, don't see how I can possess it." He put the order in his pocket. "Sorry to trouble you gentlemen," he apologized, a mischievous twinkle in his eyes.

"That's all right, Sheriff," Nightingale sympathized. "Can't blame you for doing your duty." He winked broadly at me. "Gotta rush back to Decatur. Take care of my car 'til I get back, will you, Harry?"

Unfortunately there was no way we could stop the legal vultures from stripping the clinic to the bone. They carted off the furniture and medical equipment, even moved beds out from under patients. Dr. Washburn, who'd stayed with me for two years in spite of all kinds of pressure by the AMA, sadly took his license off the wall and went home.

The day the clinic closed I received a phone call from my sister Nora. Will and Dan Hoxsey had driven in from Girard and wanted to see me. Shortly after dinner I dropped in at the McClughan house.

"Hear they busted you," my brother Danny greeted me. "Well, you can always come back to the mine. The old mule is whinnyin' for you." Then, turning serious: "I come to tell you I'm sorry I ever let them shysters talk me into signing that complaint against you, Harry. Don't know what got into me; guess I was plain scared, what with all their threats. I was a danged fool. Like Will said all along, all they wanted was to close you down. Now that I know what their game is, I want out. Nora, get me some paper and a pen!"

He sat right down and dashed off a letter to Lawyer Templeman, notifying him that he was withdrawing from the suit.

Brother Will put his arm around my shoulder. "Don't worry, Harry, you ain't licked yet. Wait and see, none of the family will ever testify against you. We all know Dad gave you them formulas legal and proper, and Danny and I will swear to that on a stack of Bibles if the case ever comes to trial. You'll whup 'em, and whup 'em good."

That was too much for Nora. "Here, give me that pen and paper," she said. "I'm going to quit that suit too." She did, and during the next few weeks campaigned vigorously to get the rest of the family to do likewise.

Meanwhile several of the patients who had been taking treatment at the clinic when it closed begged me to continue treating them privately. I knew my enemies were watching me like hawks, ready to pounce down on me at the slightest excuse, that I was leaving myself wide open to attack by applying the treatment without medical supervision. But at the moment no doctor dared associate himself with me, lest he too be dragged into court as party to the suit. What was I to do, let these unfortunates die?

Sure enough, within 18 months three separate complaints charging me with practicing medicine without a license were sworn out against me. I pleaded guilty to all of them, was fined $100 and costs on each charge, paid up with a clear conscience and no regrets. And I kept right on treating my patients.

In August 1929 the pretrial hearing on the suit for trover was held before Judge Thomas Jett, one of the most venerable and respected jurists in the state. The plaintiffs were represented by Attorney Templeman, with the assistance of the two lawyers from Chicago. My counsel was headed by John Greer, former district attorney and county judge (and incidentally a law associate of Judge Jett before he was elected to the bench).

When I arrived in Court that Monday morning I found two of my attorneys waiting for me, but Judge Greer hadn't come in yet. On the table were the briefs we were going to file—three of them, each at least two inches thick, citing all kinds of cases bearing on the question of trover. I glanced nervously at my watch, court was due to open in 15 minutes and my chief counsel hadn't arrived.

A few minutes later he strolled in, took a seat at our table, and pushed the briefs aside. "We don't need these," he said. Reaching into his breast pocket he pulled out a single sheet of legal paper and laid it on the table. "This is our brief," he announced. I read it quickly, over his shoulder.

It was a petition asking for dismissal of the charges on the grounds of common law. In support, it cited two cases about 100 years old. The first dealt with the rights to a patent on a maple syrup cooker developed by two partners in Vermont. The business failed, and the partnership was dissolved. When one of the partners set up another business and successfully promoted the same cooker, he was sued for a share of the profits. The court held for the defendant.

The other case was tried in New Hampshire. It dealt with the rights to a patent formerly held by a machine tool company that went bankrupt. One of the partners took up the same patent and was so successful with it that within a few years he was able to pay off all the debts of the bankrupt company. The other partner promptly

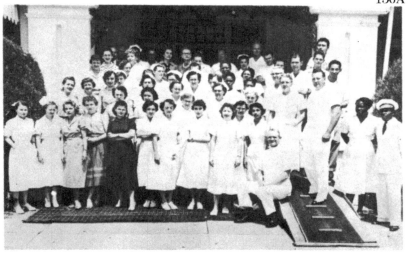

The staff of the Hoxsey Cancer Clinic at Dallas, Texas. Among the 60 employes are 7 doctors, 26 nurses, 8 x-ray technicians and 5 laboratory technicians.

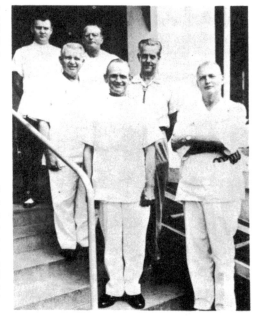

Doctors at the Clinic are (first row) Dr. Benjamin A. Harry and Dr. Douglas C. Logan; (second row) Dr. Alfred H. Staffa and Dr. Donald Watt; (back row) Dr. Charles P. Barberee and Dr. William E. Stokes. Not shown is Dr. Walter F. Pickett, M.D., who recently joined the staff.

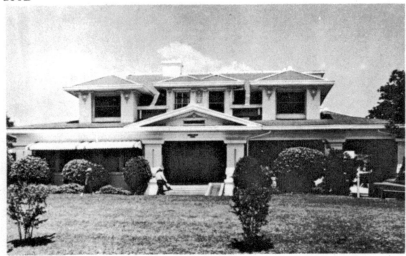

The Hoxsey Cancer Clinic—a 60 room converted residence about a mile from the heart of downtown Dallas.

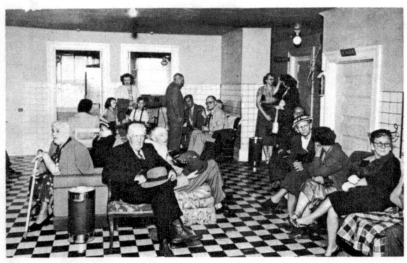

Patients from all over the country await their turn for examination and various clinical tests.

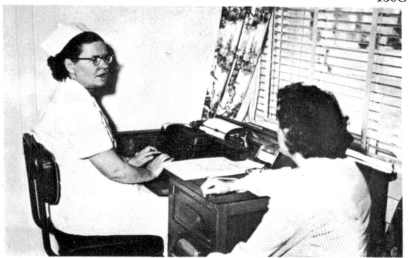

The routine for new patients begins with an interview by a nurse who takes down a complete medical history.

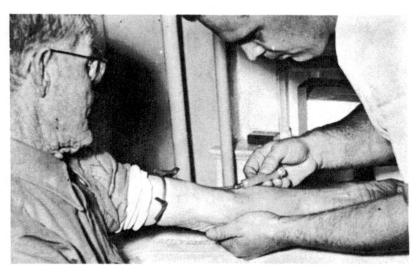

Laboratory tests include blood count and analysis, urinalysis, bacteriological tests, etc.

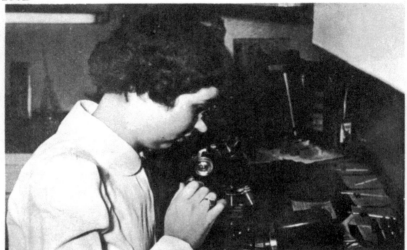

The Clinic in Dallas maintains two fully equipped laboratories staffed by trained, competent technicians.

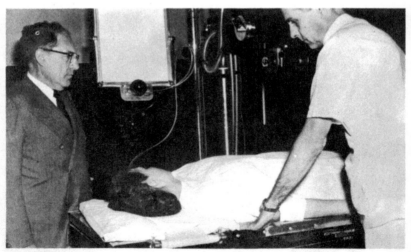

A licensed roentgenologist takes a full series of x-ray photographs of each patient.

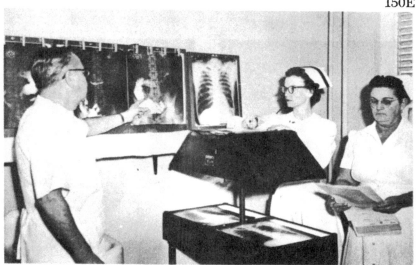

The x-ray photos go up on a battery of reading boxes, later are studied in the steroscopic viewer.

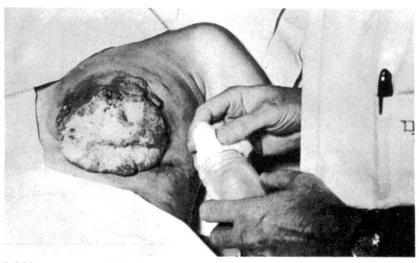

A hideous cancer of the breast is treated with the Hoxsey external medicines.

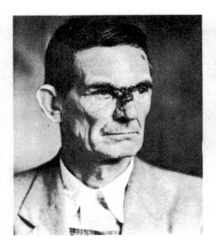
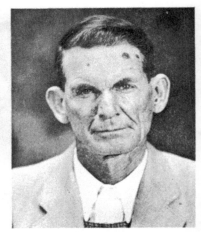

A. J. Atkinson of Wilmer, Texas. Photo at left was taken Dec. 29, 1937; at right, Feb. 12, 1938.

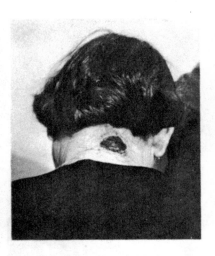
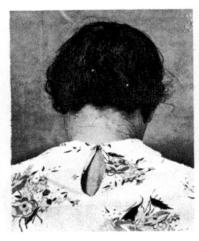

Mrs. J. A. Raub of Wichita Falls, Texas. Photo at left, Nov. 15, 1937; at right, Jan. 8, 1939.

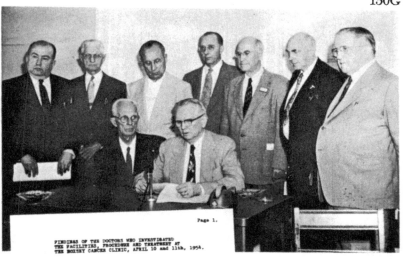

Page 1.

FINDINGS OF THE DOCTORS WHO INVESTIGATED
THE FACILITIES, PROCEDURE AND TREATMENT AT
THE HOXSEY CANCER CLINIC, APRIL 10 and 11th, 1954.

The Br   ? ~~ ~~ton Avenue, De````

interrogating former patients and going over hundreds of charts,
case histories, x-ray films, medical histories and biopsy reports.
We find as a fact that our investigation has demonstrated to
our satisfaction that the Hoxsey Cancer Clinic at Dallas, Texas
is successfully treating pathologically proven cases of cancer,
both internal and external without the use of surgery, radium
or x-ray. Accepting the standard yard-stick of cases that
have remained symptom-free in excess of five to six years
after treatment, established by medical authorities, we have
seen sufficient cases to warrant such a conclusion. Some of
those presented before us have been free of symptoms as long
as twenty-four years, and the physical evidence indicates that
they are all enjoying exceptional health at this time.

We as a committee, feel that the Hoxsey treatment is superior
to such conventional methods of treatment as x-ray, radium
and surgery. We are willing to assist this clinic in any way
possible in bringing this treatment to the American public. We
are willing to use it in our office, in our practice on our own
patients when, at our discretion it is deemed necessary.
The above statement represents the unanimous findings of this
committee. In testimony thereunto we hereby attach our
signatures.

Last year 10 M.D.'s who investigated the Hoxsey treatment declared it successful and "superior to conventional methods." Here is their signed statement, as read by their spokesman, Dr. E. E. Loffler of Spokane, Wash.

April 12, 1954.

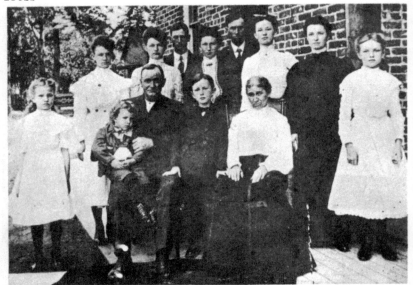

The Hoxsey family in 1904. Eleven of the 12 children appear, with Harry on his father's lap.

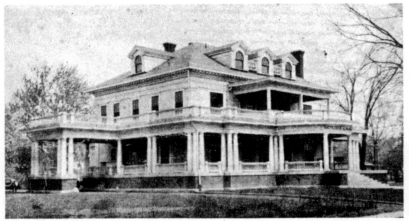

The Hoxide Cancer Sanitarium, one of the landmarks of Taylorville, Ill. in 1924.

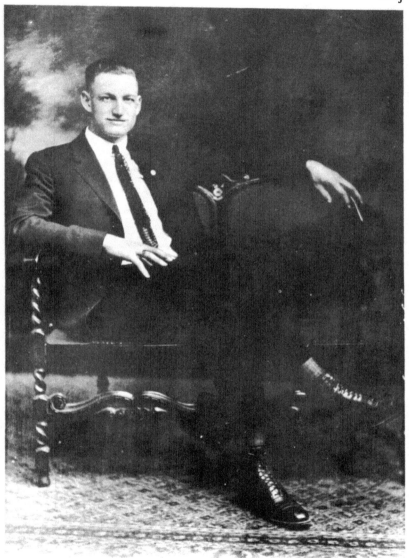

Harry M. Hoxsey at the age of 21, when cancer patients first came to him, looking for a miracle.

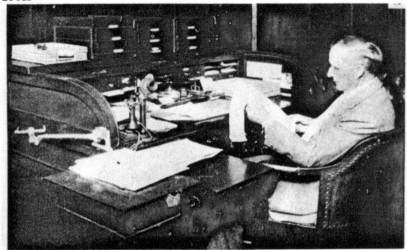

Dr. George H. Simmons. Organized medicine in America was his creation, and remains his memorial.

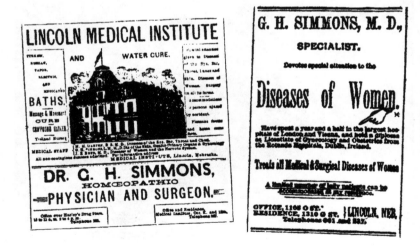

These ads appeared in newspapers of Lincoln, Neb. several years before Simmons got his mail-order degree (Chapter 8).

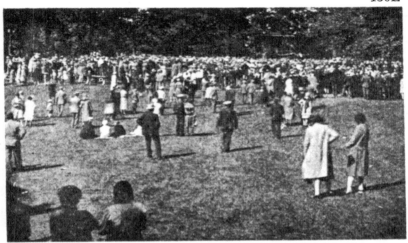

32,000 people turned out in a demonstration at Muscatine, Iowa on May 30, 1930, to witness the "resurrection" of Mandus Johnson (Chapter 11). Cancer covered entire top of his skull (left). Fully healed (right) he lived on for 30 years.

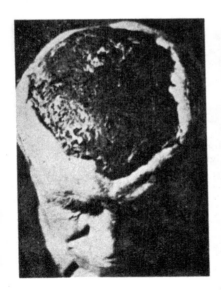

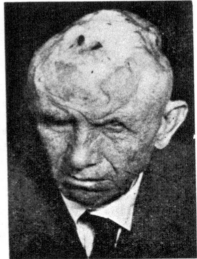

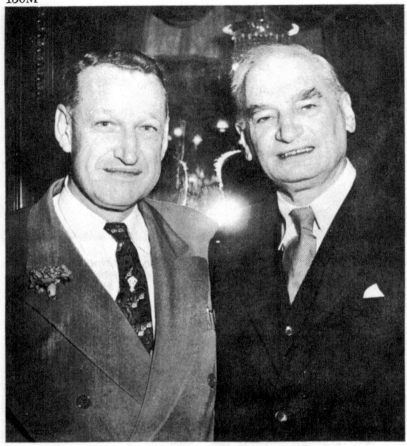

Harry M. Hoxsey with U.S. Senator William Langer, after latter introduced bill for Congressional investigation of treatment.

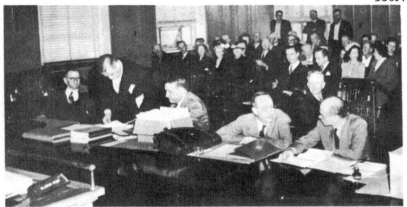

Counsel table at trial of libel and slander suit vs. Hearst (Chapter 15). Bending over table beside Hoxsey is his principal counsel, Herbert Hyde.

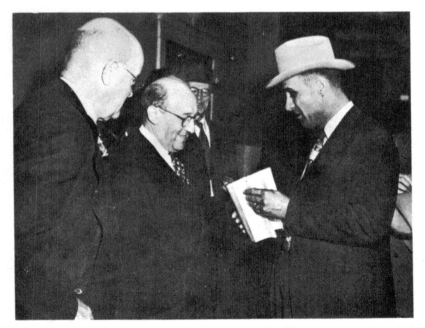

Dr. Morris Fishbein, "surprise" witness in the Hearst case, is handed summons to defend himself against libel and slander charges.

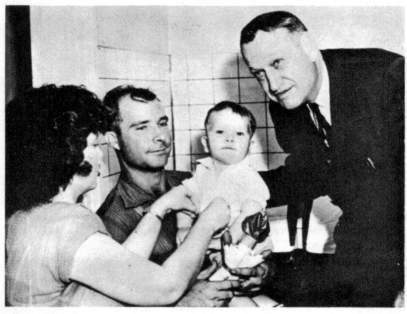

Doctors who operated on 5-week-old John Wayne Seago (above with parents and Hoxsey) said his case was hopeless. Now 2½ years old, except for scar on abdomen (right) he shows no trace of ordeal.

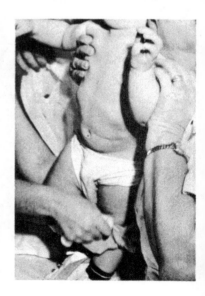

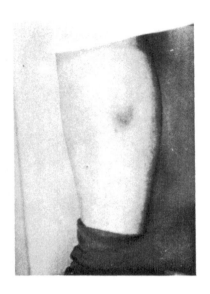

Melanocarcinoma on leg of Mildred Rager, successfully treated at Hoxsey Clinic. (Below) Clifton H. Smith tells (Chapter 17) how Hoxsey treatment cured him of cancer.

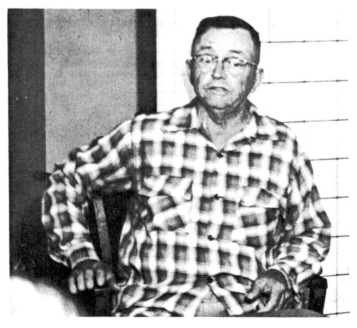

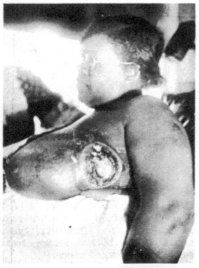 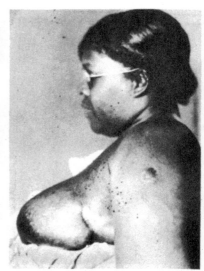

Mrs. Ethel Dennis of Philadelphia, treated for cancer of the breast in 1934 (Chapter 12). Before and after treatment. Biopsy report below, from well-known laboratory, attests that this patient had cancer when our treatment began.

LELAND BROWN LABORATORIES
422 CENTER BUILDING
6916 MARKET STREET
UPPER DARBY, PA.

PHONE, BOULEVARD 4838

June 27, 1934.

Dr. E. M. Hewish,
2131 Columbia Ave.,
Philadelphia, Pa.

Dear Mr. Hewish,

Examination of piece of tissue, taken from breast of Mrs. Dennis, 2040 Turner Street, Philadelphia shows the presence of cords of cancer cells arranged in rows with infiltration of the cells into the surrounding tissue. The stratified squamous epithelium is intact.

DIAGNOSIS: Tubular carcinoma.

Very truly yours,

LELAND BROWN LABORATORIES,

By: *[signature]* M.D.

Pathologist.

sued for a share of the profits. The Court held for the defendant; it said that the plaintiff was free to exploit the same patent separately, if he wished, but he couldn't prevent his former partner from also exploiting it. Nor was he entitled to a share of his former partner's new business.

My other lawyers were incredulous. "John, you mean you want us to throw away the legal briefs we've worked on all these months and use only this? This isn't a brief, it's just a petition!"

Judge Greer nodded. "I mean exactly that. The petition cites parallel cases, and they fit us like a glove. The main issue involved in each decision cited—namely the rights of the plaintiff to a share in the proceeds of a property he once abandoned—is identical with the main issue of the case we're trying. That issue has been decided before. Therefore we want the case dismissed. That's all there is to this case. There's nothing more to say. As to its length, let me remind you that Abe Lincoln never wrote a brief longer than 5 pages, and he had a habit of winning his cases!"

"But these are at least 100 years old," they objected.

Greer smiled. "That's what makes them common law. Do you think the common law on trover has changed during the past 100 years? As you know, a rule of common law can be abolished only by express statute. I've looked all through the statute books, and there's no law or decision which invalidates the decisions we cite here."

At that moment the clerk sharply rapped his gavel, Judge Jett appeared and took his place on the bench. When our case was announced, Judge Greer got up and addressed the bench.

"Your Honor, instead of a brief, we'd like to submit a petition to the Honorable Court. It is exactly one page long, and cites only two cases. I believe these two cases should help resolve the issue before us." He passed the paper up to the bench.

Judge Jett frowned, put on his glasses and read slowly, his head moving from side to side, his lips moving slightly as he digested the contents. As he read the frown slowly evaporated from his face, was replaced by a benign smile.

"These are pretty old cases, Mr. Greer," he said mildly. "I'd like to see the reports you refer to. I wonder where such old reports can be found in a town like this."

John walked back to the counsel table, hefted his brief case to a chair, unstrapped it and pulled out two large tomes, yellow with age. Opening each at a marker, he took them to the bench and carefully handed them to the judge.

Again Judge Jett's head moved from side to side, his lips silently formed words. He finished one report, laid it aside, read the other. Concluding it, he took a sip of water, thoughtfully polished his spectacles and put them back on his nose.

"Let me congratulate you, Mr. Greer," he said. "I think these cases are very much to the point. And I can't see what counsel for the complainant can show to invalidate that point. So I am going to grant your petition!"

Attorney Templeman was on his feet. "Your honor," he protested, "we're waiting for another attorney to appear and present our brief in this case. We feel we are entitled to a hearing."

"I see no reason why we should waste the time of the court adjudicating a case that is as clear as this one, Mr.

Templeman," Judge Jett said firmly. He signed the petition.

As we enthusiastically pumped Judge Greer's hand, one of my lawyers demanded: "Where on earth did you dig those old-timers up, John?"

"I didn't," Greer said, with a broad grin. "They were dug up for me on condition that I never tell who did the digging. So don't ask me any more questions."

I opened one of the ancient books of reports. On the fly-leaf were the words: *"From the library of Thomas Jett."*

During the victory celebration at my house that evening, my brother Danny suddenly turned to me and said: "Something about Judge Jett nagged me all through the hearing, and I just couldn't put my finger on it. Now it's come to me. I met him before, a long time ago."

"Where?"

"At our house in Girard. You wouldn't remember, you were just a little fellow then. He came with his step-aunt, who lived in the valley beyond Round Tree. Dad was treating her for cancer of the insides. Two doctors told her she was going to die of it, but our Daddy cured her. She lived 10 or 12 years after that."

A big smile on his face, he added: "She raised Tom Jett from the time he was knee-high; both his parents were dead, it was her money put him through college. And he fair worshipped her!"

A "Persecution Complex"?

IT WAS a legal and moral victory, but an extremely costly one. The fine clinic I'd put over with so much sweat and struggle was gone. Moreover the nuisance suit had cost me at least $88,000 in expense and financial loss. By the time it wound up I was flat broke, virtually penniless.

I needed money for a new clinic, but was reluctant to appeal for help to friends in Taylorville who'd stood by me so staunchly thus far in my knock-down, drag-out battle with the AMA—a battle that I knew was just beginning.

The problem was solved when a group of prominent citizens in Girard offered me financial backing if I'd return to my old home town and set up practice there.

We bought the old Nicolet Hotel, converted it into a cancer clinic and hospital. Dr. Miller, once more in complete accord with my policies, agreed to come down from Chicago every week and supervise the treatment of patients. The day the clinic opened—July 17, 1929—was designated "Hoxsey Day" by the Girard Chamber of Commerce, and it sponsored a giant demonstration in which the entire countryside turned out to hear numerous speakers—including former patients, local officials and even some doctors—testify to the efficiency of the Hoxsey treatment.

154

I frequently had been accused of being a flamboyant showman and promoter, as well as a healer.

If I am all these things, it is because the AMA forced these roles upon me. The relentless campaign of innuendo and outright slander against me and my treatment has been largely a subterranean one. As history indicates, the medical hierarchy always has shunned the light of public discussion and investigation in any professional controversy. I had to find some way to get my cases before the public and promote what my enemies were anxiously avoiding—a public showdown on the true merits of the Hoxsey treatment.

The plain truth is, I had to become both showman and promoter in order to continue to treat cancer by unorthodox methods and survive.

Ironically enough my unceasing effort to turn the spotlight on a controversy in which the public is vitally concerned has been cited by the self-appointed guardians of professional morals as proof that I am an "unethical quack."

To the AMA, ethics are more precious than human life! The bankruptcy of the charge is obvious. Publicity is the friend of truth, the enemy of fraud and deceit. No quack willingly lays his head down on the public block and begs his enemies to chop it off. I have done so repeatedly during the past 30 years. And my head is still intact on my shoulders.

Before opening my new clinic I offered Dr. Morris Fishbein, editor of the AMA *Journal,* another chance with the hatchet. We sent him an invitation urging him to attend the celebration, get a first-hand look at our method of treating cancer, and state his conclusions in public.

There was no direct response. Instead about three weeks later his *Journal* came out with another blast at the Hoxsey treatment. Doctors began to tell my patients that I was a "notorious quack." My reply was—still is— that I'd rather be notorious, and save people's lives, than famous and bury them.

Because we did save lives our clinic prospered, and its reputation gradually spread throughout the Middle West.

One day in February 1930 I received a long distance telephone call from Norman G. Baker, who operated a hospital at Muscatine, Iowa. He said his doctors had been experimenting with various cancer treatments and weren't satisfied with the results. He'd had excellent reports on my treatment from Dr. Charles L. Loffler of Chicago. Would I be willing to come to Muscatine and demonstrate my treatment?

I'd heard of Baker and his hospital before; both were widely publicized throughout the Middle West in daily broadcasts from his own radio station, KTNT. Although he was not an M.D., and his institution didn't have the AMA seal of approval, the doctors employed there were duly licensed to practice medicine in the State of Iowa. I was more than willing to demonstrate my treatment to any doctors anywhere, at any time. Because after 10 years of treating and curing cancer in Girard and Taylorville, I felt it was high time that this treatment—with or without the sanction of organized medicine—be made available to millions of other hopeless and helpless cancer victims throughout the nation.

So I got into my car the next morning, and arrived at Muscatine that same afternoon.

Norman Baker turned out to be a handsome, wavy-haired, middle-aged, aggressive personality with hypnotic eyes. Indeed he had once made a living as a hypnotist on the vaudeville stage, and had married Eva Tanguay, the famous "I Don't Care" girl of the early '20s. When I told him about my difficulties with the AMA he replied that he didn't give a damn about the medical bureaucracy, all he was interested in was results. He called in his chief of staff, Dr. Statler; after an hour's discussion I agreed to show what I could do.

We went through the hospital, selected 25 cancer cases and I administered my treatment to them. That evening in a broadcast from station KTNT I told the story of my treatment, described some of the cases I'd just taken on, announced that I would return the following Monday and treat 100 more cases of cancer.

On the appointed day I found more than 300 patients waiting for me at the hospital. I treated 50 of them that day. During the next few weeks, commuting regularly between Girard and Muscatine, I treated no fewer than 50 new cases of cancer per day. The rapid recovery before their very eyes of numerous patients hitherto considered hopeless astounded Dr. Statler and his colleagues, and they enthusiastically endorsed my treatment.

Baker called me in and made me a proposition. If I'd give up my own clinic and devote my full time and attention to his institution, he'd expand its facilities and convert it into the greatest cancer clinic and hospital in the world. He'd put in the most modern equipment money could buy, staff it with the most competent professional and technical help available, launch a tremendous publicity campaign to make the treatment known to cancer sufferers all over the nation. His doctors would cooperate with me 100 percent, and he would back me to the limit in any further conflict with the AMA.

The glowing picture he painted was extremely tempting, but I was very hesitant about accepting his proposition. I'd seen and heard enough about him to realize that he was a shrewd operator, interested primarily in personal profit. And this recalled disagreeably my experience six years before with Everhard and his money-hungry associates.

I informed Baker that the basic principle I'd always maintained—low fees and free treatment for charity cases —must be continued in the new enterprise or I wanted no part in it. This policy wasn't just altruism, I explained earnestly, it was common-sense business. The cases we cured for free were our best advertisement; they would spread the word among their neighbors, send us scores of cases who were able and willing to pay a reasonable fee for saving their lives.

After numerous discussions he finally agreed to follow this policy. Thereupon I closed my clinic at Girard and moved to Muscatine.

From the very start Norman Baker proved to be a super-salesman and past master in the art of promotion and showmanship. Day and night Station KTNT beamed the news that cancer was being successfully treated at this hospital into the homes of millions of radio listeners. He issued and distributed widely a monthly magazine devoted to the case histories and pictures of patients we'd treated. At regular intervals he'd stage public demonstrations in which patients successfully treated at our institution appeared and told their stories.

The result was a great flood of cancer sufferers from

all parts of the nation. They poured into Muscatine by train, car or bus, filled hotels, overflowed into boarding houses and private homes, jammed the waiting rooms and corridors of the hospital. Soon our over-worked doctors were treating as many as 300 cases per day.

One of the earliest and most spectacular cases treated during this period was Mandus Johnson of Galesburg, Illinois. When I first saw him on March 2, 1930 the entire top of his head was covered with a cancer (the biopsy had been made by a Dr. Baird of Galesburg). It had consumed the entire scalp, exposing the skull. Two drain tubes had been inserted into holes cut in the skull, and from these more than a pint of pus was drained every day. To this day it remains the worst case of cancer I have ever seen.

"Either cure me or kill me!" he begged. "I can't stand the odor, I'd rather be dead than like this." I had to tell him there wasn't but one chance in a million that he would survive. However I agreed to try.

Five weeks later I went on the radio and announced that the following night (April 8th) we would remove the top of Johnson's skull, and the cancer with it. People came as far as 800 miles to witness the operation. When Dr. Rasmussen and I lifted the cancer from the sick man's head, exposing the brain, 14 people in the audience fainted.

The AMA *Journal* immediately published a vicious attack upon us, asserting that Johnson had died as the result of our treatment. We quickly spiked that lie. On Decoration Day (May 30th) the "dead man" made a personal appearance—with over 100 other patients—at a giant demonstration in Weed Park, Muscatine. In the crowd of 32,000 (by actual count) that witnessed this miraculous "resurrection of the dead," and heard this modern Lazarus testify to the efficacy of the Hoxsey treatment, were more than 50 doctors. Mandus Johnson lived on, spectacular proof that we cure cancer. He died only about 5 years ago.

My association with Norman Baker lasted exactly 5 months and 20 days. As the influx of patients and cash receipts mounted (we were taking in as much as $10,000 per day from cancer cases) so did his greed and avarice. The staff and facilities of his hospital were entirely inadequate to handle the vast increase in patient load, but he refused to fulfill his promise to expand facilities, add equipment and hire more help. Instead, conceiving a crafty scheme to increase income and simultaneously solve the overload problem without additional expense, he began to demand between $750 and $1200 per case from patients, and to refuse treatment to those unwilling or unable to pay the steep tariff.

Outraged by this unscrupulous violation of our agreement, I protested that the country was in the midst of a serious business depression; millions were unemployed and could scarcely keep food in the mouths of their families, let alone pay medical expenses. Were we going to let these people die? His callous reply was: "When it's a matter of life or death, people always manage to dig up the cash!"

I put on my hat and coat and went home. And a few days later Norman Baker went on the air to announce a "new, improved treatment guaranteed to cure all types of cancer."

(His new treatment proved worthless, the Federal

Communications Commission took away his broadcasting license, local pressure forced him to move his hospital first to Laredo, Texas, then to Eureka Springs, Arkansas. He continued to broadcast from station XENT, just across the border from Del Rio, Texas. Justice finally caught up with him ten years later. I was subpoenaed by the Government and testified at his trial at Little Rock, Arkansas. On January 23, 1940, he was convicted of using the mails to defraud, fined $4,000, and sentenced to four years in Leavenworth. Released in July 1944, he retired to Florida to live a life of luxury on a yacht.)

Organized medicine has made much of my short-lived association with Baker. It completely ignores the fact that relentless persecution by the AMA made it impossible for me at that time to obtain more reputable collaborators. I had no alternative. If the Devil himself had offered me the facilities and doctors to treat cancer legitimately, and thus save the lives of thousands of victims, I would have accepted. The moment he violated the principles I've always maintained, tried to turn my treatment into a racket, our paths would part. So it was with Baker. My brief association with him is more than justified by the fact that countless human beings who otherwise might be dead and buried are still alive and healthy today.

In conjunction with Dr. Rasmussen and my cousin, Dr. T. T. Hoxsey, M.D., I opened a new clinic at Muscatine and continued to give cancer victims the Hoxsey treatment, whether they could afford it or not.

Soon after our new clinic opened a Capt. Larsen of Detroit, Michigan heard about us and paid us a visit. Greatly impressed by what he saw and heard, on his return home he called on his friend Ernest A. Maross and told him the story of the Hoxsey treatment. Maross was a figure of considerable substance and standing in the automobile industry; he'd helped finance Henry Ford in his early experiments, was one of the founders of the Indianapolis Speedway and a leading importer of foreign racing cars. His interest in cancer was more than academic; a close relative recently had been stricken by the dread disease.

Maross came out to Muscatine to see for himself, accompanied by his wife, his brother Joe and the latter's wife, former grand opera star Maude Slocum. After observing the treatment and talking with patients, Mrs. Maross urged me to come to Detroit and found a free clinic there. She offered to finance the venture for 90 days; if in that time we could successfully treat at least 50 percent of the patients who presented themselves, she would endorse the treatment, sponsor the clinic and obtain the sponsorship of other prominent citizens—people of the caliber of Henry and Wilfred Leland, who built the Lincoln automobile, Congressman John Sosnosky, and others.

We leaped at the opportunity to knock on the head, once and for all, the AMA slander that the Hoxsey treatment was just a lucrative "racket." Certainly nothing could be less lucrative than a free, non-profit clinic supported and sponsored by reputable citizens. Perhaps, with that diversionary charge scotched, the medical profession could be induced to focus its attention on the results we were getting.

So with high hopes we closed the clinic in Muscatine and Dr. Rasmussen and I moved to Detroit.

Our new location was a 5-room suite in a large apartment building owned by Mrs. Maross on Woodward Avenue, the city's principal thoroughfare. Her personal physician, Dr. Homer B. Van Hyning, M.D., agreed to donate 90 days of his time to test the value of the treatment. We got off to a fine start. All the newspapers carried stories about the new clinic, and we announced over radio station WMEC that there would be no charge for treatment, we would accept only charity cases.

The opening of the clinic on March 8, 1931, was attended by the Marosses, the Lelands, Mary Kuney and a host of other socially prominent people. That day 118 patients were accepted for free treatment.

If we had any illusions that the AMA would call off its dogs now, they soon evaporated. There's only one thing that organized medicine fears more than unorthodoxy, and that's free medical treatment. It hits them where it hurts most—in the pocketbook. Faced with the double-barrelled threat of a free clinic dedicated to the Hoxsey method, the AMA lost no time in mobilizing its forces.

Two days after the clinic opened I was abruptly summoned to the Prosecuting Attorney's office. Ernest Maross accompanied me there. We were received by the Assistant Prosecutor Duncan M. McCrae, who informed us that his office had received a number of complaints charging me with practicing medicine illegally. I replied that I was permitted by law to treat patients under the direction of a qualified physician; Dr. Van Hyning, the medical director of our clinic, was fully licensed to practice in the State of Michigan. McCrae questioned us closely about the clinic, its operation and its financing. Then, surveying us speculatively, he observed:

"Confidentially, you boys are up against a tough proposition. The Wayne County Medical Society is out to bust you, and it swings a lot of political weight. You need good legal advice. Now if you were to pay me $200 a week, I'm sure you wouldn't have any further trouble with this office—"

Dumbfounded by this brazen shakedown, Maross and I just looked at each other. He shook his head, and we got up. "You can go plumb to hell," I said evenly. We walked out.

(In this connection it is interesting to note that a few years later Duncan McCrae was convicted of taking graft and running a "protection" racket in the Prosecutor's office. He was sent to the State Penitentiary and served time for this crime.)

The payoff came ten days later when I was arrested on a formal charge of practicing medicine without a license. Maross immediately put up bail and provided me with three excellent attorneys, Carl M. Weideman, Max Marston and Peter J. Drexcelius.

We went to trial on May 8th in Recorder's Court, Detroit, before Judge W. McKay Skillman. The State's brief was presented by our old friend and would-be protector, Asst. Pros. Atty. Duncan McCrae. And as soon as his principal witness took the stand, I knew that the case against me had been carefully framed by experts.

The day the clinic opened this same individual, posing as a patient, had come in and asked to see "Dr. Hoxsey." He was told that Mr. Hoxsey was not a doctor, but a medical technician. Interviewed by Dr. Van Hyning, he stated that he was in severe pain, and that several doctors had diagnosed his trouble as cancer of the stomach and bowels. Thorough examination disclosing no sign of cancer, Dr. Van Hyning advised the alleged patient that he was suffering from nothing more serious than colitis and sent him home.

Now he identified himself as Otto Fischl, investigator for the State Medical Board, and unfolded a much more colorful account of his experiences at the clinic. He declared that he was examined by both Dr. Van Hynin and me, that we held a conference in *"something that sounded like Latin,"* that he heard me say (in good English, this time): *"No, it is a cancer!"* The doctor then informed him: *"You have something far more worse than cancer, you have tumors around your intestines."* He further testified that I gave him some pills and medicine, and when he offered to pay told him: *"It doesn't cost you anything now. We'll find out later how you feel. Come back next week."*

Sharp cross-examination failed to shake his story, although he amended it slightly by conceding: *"Mr. Hoxsey didn't tell me what was wrong with me then, nor did he tell me at any time."* He also admitted: *"To the best of my knowledge there was nothing to indicate to me that Mr. Hoxsey was a doctor."*

The State's only other witness, an elderly lady named Mrs. Rowena Barr, at once demonstrated that although she'd been subpoenaed she didn't want any part in this legal lynching. When McCrae asked her if she was a patient at the clinic, she retorted:

"Indeed I am, and they've cured me!"

Dazed by this unexpected blow, the Prosecutor led with his chin by asking how she knew she had cancer. The sharp return rocked him back on his heels:

"My own doctor told me so. He said I'm going to die of it!" She tried to get the physician's name into the record (he was a very prominent specialist) but McCrae had taken enough punishment.

"No more questions," he snapped.

Whereupon the sweet little old lady sniffed loudly: *"This looks more like persecution than prosecution!"* The spectators broke into loud laughter and applause, the judge banged his gavel and threatened to clear the courtroom.

When our turn came both Dr. Van Hyning and I declared under oath that Fischl's story was entirely false. (In fact I cannot speak Latin. Never had time to learn that language, or any other except English.) And during the next three days more than 80 patients took the stand to testify that they owed their lives to our clinic and that we never charged them a cent for treatment.

Yet after a most vicious harangue by Prosecutor McCrae and a particularly prejudicial charge by Judge Skillman, the jury of 7 women and 5 men returned a verdict of guilty!

Urging that the verdict was contrary to the evidence, my attorneys at once filed a motion for a new trial. On Saturday May 18th the motion was denied, and Judge Skillman sentenced me to 6 months in jail and a $200 fine.

We immediately announced we would appeal, and Ernest Maross offered to put up a $5,000 cash bond for my appearance. McCrae maliciously told him it was too late, the courthouse and Prosecutor's office had already closed for the weekend. So I was forced to spend the weekend in the Wayne County jail. Early Monday morning Maross appeared to make bond—and discovered it couldn't be accepted because the Prosecutor in charge of the case had gone on vacation! I would have to spend the next two weeks in jail! Weary of this run-around, my attorneys applied for a writ of habeas corpus. Apprised of this move, McCrae suddenly turned up and approved my bond. I finally was released.

It took nearly 17 months to get action on our appeal. On Dec. 6, 1932, the Michigan State Supreme Court, by unanimous decision of all 8 Justices on the bench, reversed the conviction:

> "The physician, according to the testimony, had charge of the case and the assistance given the physician by defendant did not constitute practicing the profession of physician. The charges were not established and the conviction is reversed and defendant discharged."

Baldly implying prejudice on the part of Judge Skillman, the Justices went out of their way to spank him in these words:

> "Defendant's motion for a new trial pointed out that the proofs did not establish any violation of law, and the motion should have been granted."

I was completely vindicated, my right to treat cancer under the supervision of a qualified doctor was fully established. But in the interval between conviction and vindication the AMA had gained its principal objective. The State Medical Board revoked Dr. Van Hyning's license to practice in Michigan, he retired to a small town in Ohio, and no other doctor with guts enough to buck the powerful combination could be found.

The free clinic was forced to close.

Whenever spokesmen for the AMA are confronted with the charge that this organization has conspired continuously to suppress my treatment, their stock answer is that I suffer from a "persecution complex."

As official records in several cities will show, any "complex" I may have is more than justified by the relentless persecution I have suffered.

Of Mice—and Men

In May 1932, while my appeal in Michigan was still pending I entered into a contract with Dr. J. R. Arnold, well-known surgeon at Wheeling, West Virginia, to establish a clinic in that city.

Instantly the County Medical Society stepped in with a repetition of the tactics used so successfully against us by its colleagues in Detroit. While we were still remodelling our offices, before a single patient could be examined or treated, I was arrested on a charge of illegal practice of medicine. Bail was set at $10,000, an excessive amount for the misdemeanor with which I was charged. It was immediately supplied by two friends, C. M. Watson and S. K. Frank.

I returned to our offices and proceeded with the remodelling. We made arrangements for a 15-minute broadcast every day from station WWVA, whose studios adjoined our clinic. The State Medical Society informed the station that if we were permitted to broadcast it would file a complaint with the FCC in Washington, demanding that the station's broadcasting license be revoked. In the face of this threat, WWVA cancelled our contract.

At the hearing in the Justice of Peace court, Dr. Arnold declared that he was to be medical director of the clinic, and that I would have nothing whatsoever to do with examination, treatment or prescriptions. Nevertheless upon the insistence of the Prosecutor I was placed under $1,000 bond for appearance before the Grand Jury, two months hence.

Throughout these 60 days Dr. Arnold was harassed and hounded and threatened with loss of his license by the local Medical Society. Finally he came to me and said he couldn't take the pressure, he was forced to discontinue his connection with the clinic. And that was that.

Two weeks after the clinic closed the Grand Jury heard the evidence in the case against me, and refused to indict. I was free, but there was no further reason to remain in Wheeling.

During a much-needed vacation in Atlantic City I met Dr. Willard M. Mason, a local physician, and Al Perkins, the local postmaster. Both were intensely interested in my account of the Hoxsey treatment. Perkins told me about his friend Howard Hickman, who had a bad cancer on his face.

"If you can cure him," the postmaster declared, "I'll see to it that you open a clinic here and are not bothered by the law." Dr. Mason agreeing to supervise treatment, I accepted the challenge.

They brought Hickman to the post office and I treated him right in the private office of the postmaster. The next day they brought in a man named Clarence Parker who had a cancer that covered most of his nose, and I treated him too. After a few weeks the cancers disappeared from the faces of both these men.

Convinced by this demonstration that I could cure cancer, Dr. Mason proposed that we open a clinic at his home on South Ventnor Avenue in Atlantic City. I accepted.

One of our first patients was Capt. Richard Higby, a former merchant marine skipper and father of the Atlantic City Chief of Police. Capt. Higby had a cancer that covered his nose and had spread to both eyes and the forehead. We treated him, and cured him.

Shortly thereafter the attorney for the local County Medical Society applied for a warrant for my arrest. He was sent to see Chief of Police Higby. That official bluntly told him: "Hoxsey saved my father's life. If you dare to lay a finger on him, I personally will see to it that every one of you goes to jail for false arrest. Now get the hell out of my office!"

For the remainder of my stay in Atlantic City I was not molested.

In March, 1933, one of my sponsors, Hazen G. Kniffin, arranged a meeting with Dr. George Dorrance of the Oncological Cancer Hospital in Philadelphia. Dr. Dorrance spent more than two hours inspecting the case histories, medical records and photographs we presented. Then he suggested that Dr. Mason and I bring ten patients in various stages of treatment to the hospital in Philadelphia so that a group of doctors could examine them, determine whether they actually had cancer and observe their reactions to our treatment.

We put 15 patients into three automobiles and drove to Philadelphia. At the hospital Dr. Dorrance, Dr. B. A. Hughes and some 20 other members of the staff examined each patient, carefully went over our medical records and declared that the evidence was very impressive. Would we treat 25 charity cases, under their supervision? We readily accepted and were told to come back the following week, at which time the patients would be made available to us.

On our return to Atlantic City we told Judge Joseph Thompson, a banker and former Mayor of the city, of the arrangements we'd just made. His son recently had died of cancer, so he was very much interested. Moreover, he knew Dr. Dorrance personally. He picked up the telephone, called Dr. Dorrance, and obtained permission to watch the experiment.

The following week Judge Thompson picked us up—Dr. Mason, Kniffen, their friend Capt. Cooksen and myself—in his luxurious car and his chauffeur drove us to Philadelphia. Dr. Dorrance met us at the door to the hospital. He said he'd been in touch with the AMA; before I could treat any patient at his hospital I'd have to give him my formulas in writing. Recalling my experience with Dr. Harris, I refused. However I offered a compromise:

"Let me treat these 25 patients. If they get well, and you officially state that my treatment cured them, I'll release my formulas to the entire medical profession."

He repeated that he had to have the formulas first. Judge Thompson urged him to accept my offer; after all there were 25 human lives at stake. The good doctor replied:

"Twenty-five more or less makes little difference. We lose them by the hundreds here!"

Obviously nothing could be accomplished there. We got into the car and returned to Atlantic City.

A few weeks later Dr. Ira W. Drew, for 20 years professor of children's diseases at the Philadelphia Osteo-

pathic College, visited our clinic. He came at the request
of S. S. Preston, a wealthy patient who'd lost his wife to
cancer. Dr. Drew remained for several days, observing
our methods and examining patients in various stages of
treatment. At the end of that time he told me:

"Organized medicine will never accept you, Hoxsey.
We osteopaths have had plenty of experience with the
medical monopoly. They've fought us tooth and nail for
40 years, trying to keep us from practicing medicine.
Even though our training is as thorough as that of any
other doctor, and in most states we are now admitted to
practice on a par with other doctors, they still insist
we're not legitimate physicians, bar us from the staff of
approved hospitals. You're just wasting your time trying
to get them to recognize your treatment.

"Why don't you come to Philadelphia, work with me
and my wife" (she too was an osteopathic physician) "at
our clinic? It's a big city, you'll meet osteopaths from all
over the county and have a chance to show them what
you can do. The AMA can't touch us, scare us or buy us
off. I promise you I'll fight this thing through with you to
the bitter end."

I discussed this proposal with Dr. Mason and he advised me to accept. So I moved to Philadelphia, went to
live at the Drew home and worked at the Drew Clinic on
Wayne Avenue, in Germantown.

The black depression was in full swing, and that Spring
(1933) it reached the lowest point in history. Nearly
2500 banks all over the nation had shut their doors, wip-
ing out the life savings of millions of depositors. There
were 15 million unemployed; more than 4½ million
American families had sunk so low that in order to keep

body and soul together they had to accept public relief of one kind or another. Although the relentless tide of cancer had risen to a new high, people couldn't afford expensive surgery, x-ray and radium, many were sent home to die without treatment.

More than 90 percent of our patients at the Drew Clinic were charity cases. We took them all—rich and poor—and treated them all alike. And many recovered to see better times.

Dr. Drew enjoyed an excellent reputation, even in orthodox medical circles, and many prominent physicians attended our clinic regularly, observed our work and sent us patients. Among them were Dr. Louis B. Heimer, M.D., head of the American Stomach Hospital; Dr. E. M. Hewish, M.D., Dr. I. Sylvester Hart, D.O., and his wife, Dr. Effie Hart; Dr. Henry Bellew, D.O., and Dr. George T. Hayman, D.O.

One day, I recall, Dr. Hewish, told us he had a very serious case of breast cancer for us. The patient had been given extensive x-ray at the Philadelphia General Hospital, was badly burned but failed to show any improvement. Her name was Mrs. Ethel Dennis, and she was a colored lady. Would we treat her?

I told him at once to bring her right in. "Suffering doesn't recognize race, color or creed."

She came the following day and Dr. Drew examined her. Her left breast was enormously swollen, there was a hideous pustulant lesion giving off a horrible odor, the glands under the arm and in the neck were involved. Dr. Drew took a biopsy specimen and sent it to the Leland Brown Laboratories at Upper Darby, Pennsylvania. Back came a diagnosis of "tubular carcinoma."

After several weeks of treatment with internal tonic and the external powder and salve the entire cancerous mass dried up and fell out, clean scar tissue started to form, she was well again.

At this writing—more than 20 years later—Mrs. Dennis is still alive and healthy. There has been no recurrence of cancer. I frequently hear from her; she has sent me many patients.

Many laymen interested in cancer research heard about us, came to our clinic, were impressed by the results we were getting and tried to interest medical authorities in our work. One of them was Hubert G. Brower of the Endocrine Food Company, Union City, New Jersey. He'd been a classmate and personal friend of Dr. Clarence Cook Little, head of the world famous Roscoe B. Jackson Memorial Laboratory at Bar Harbor, Maine, managing director of the American Society for the Control of Cancer (a branch of the Rockefeller Cancer Institute) and probably the most eminent figure in American cancer research.

Brower was certain that Dr. Little would be interested in our treatment, even though it was highly controversial. For the distinguished doctor often had said: *"Adaptability and open-mindedness are essential psychological factors in the fight against cancer."*

So he got in touch with Dr. Little and persuaded him to send us 48 mice with cancer, some internal and some external, so that I could demonstrate upon them the efficacy of the Hoxsey treatment.

When the mice arrived at the Drew Clinic we found that 8 of them had died en route. We called in a number of outside doctors—among them Hewish, Heiner, Leland and the Harts—to witness the experiment. Of the 40 surviving mice more than a dozen were so feeble that it was obvious they wouldn't hold out long enough to take the treatment. We finally selected 26 of the strongest ones, gave half the internal treatment and the other half the external.

At the end of 12 weeks 10 of the mice treated internally and 6 of those treated externally were still alive, and careful examination revealed no trace of cancer in them. In fact they were so lively that they'd presented us with more than 200 baby mice!

Dr. Little was amazed and reluctant to believe us when we informed him that 13 of his cancerous mice were alive and well after taking the Hoxsey treatment. He asked us to meet him at the Harvard Club in New York City, and to bring the recovered rodents with us.

Dr. Ira Drew, Hubert Brower, and John C. Marscher (vice-president of the Philadelphia *Daily News*) accompanied me to New York for the meeting. Dr. Little met us at the Club. Scarcely waiting for introductions, he took the cage of mice from us and carefully inspected the marks on their ears and feet.

"By God, these are my mice!" he exclaimed. "How did you do it?"

I told him *I* didn't do it, the Hoxsey treatment was responsible for their remarkable recovery.

"Would you be willing to come to Bar Harbor and treat a group of mice under complete scientific controls, so that we can accurately determine the results of your treatment?" he demanded.

I assured him I would, and he said he'd let me know when the experiment was set up.

On Nov. 9, 1933, I received a telegram from Dr. Little announcing he was ready for me. Two days later I was in Bar Harbor. The following morning when I set out for the laboratory the temperature was well below zero, there was three feet of snow on the ground. Dr. Little and several associates were waiting, with 200 cancer-ridden mice.

We divided the rodents into two equal groups, one to be put under treatment, the other to remain untreated. Thus we could accurately measure the effect of my treatment. The 100 under treatment were further divided into two groups, half receiving the internal treatment and half the external.

Altogether I spent exactly a month at Bar Harbor, appearing at the laboratory every day to examine and administer treatment to my rodent patients. About 10 days after the experiment began several of the external cases began to show signs of marked improvement; the cancer dried up and in some instances sloughed off.

Dr. Little then left for a board meeting of the Rockefeller Cancer Foundation, taking with him the 13 mice treated and cured at the Drew Clinic and several of the external cases still under treatment. He returned at the end of four days, told me that no decision would be made until the experiment was concluded.

Early on the morning of Dec. 9th I arrived at the laboratory to find more than 60 of the treated mice still alive and thriving, whereas nearly all the untreated mice were dead or dying. A few minutes later Dr. Little called me into his office.

"Hoxsey," he said abruptly. "I wasn't aware of your long-standing feud with the AMA. It's just been called to my attention. We can't afford to get involved in such a controversy. Under the circumstances, I have no choice but to terminate this experiment at once."

I protested vigorously, pointing out that the results of the experiment already showed that my treatment was effective and the AMA's hostility unwarranted.

"We can't stop now," I pleaded. "Millions of human lives are at stake." He waved aside all my arguments. "You can cure all the mice this side of hell, it won't do you any good. Because your methods have alienated the medical profession, and you'll never get the cooperation of doctors in this country."

And that was his last word on the subject.

I left Bar Harbor the same day, more determined than ever to fight to the last ditch to put my treatment across. When I told Dr. Drew what had happened, he smiled and observed: "I'm not surprised. Little is a scientist with considerable prestige, but he's wise enough to know that he can't buck the medical monopoly. It's only ideal-ists like you and me who can afford that luxury. Let him play around with his mice; we'll go on treating and cur-ing human beings."

I continued working with Dr. Drew for about two years, during which time we successfully treated hun-dreds of cases of cancer, nearly all of them charity. I have before me a copy of a letter which Dr. Drew recently sent to a mutual friend, in which he states:

"During the nearly two years that Hoxsey was with me, we cared for many cases of cancer, people coming from all parts of the country. Cancers of the face, arms, legs, breast and nearly all parts of the body were presented. The results were astonishing. Many of these patients are alive and well today, more than 20 years later.

"Organized Osteopathy frowns on the Hoxsey treatment and expels members who use it from the American Osteopathic Association. But the mounting interest in this work among members of the profesion is something that cannot be ignored."

But I was getting restless. Time was moving along; I was nearly 35 years old, I'd been treating cancer for close to 15 years and yet my ultimate goal—recognition and acceptance by the medical profession—was as distant as ever. All I had to show for my troubles was an empty pocketbook, a pregnant wife and a bleak future.

Perhaps a change in scenery would help.

Early in 1936 I heard about the Spann Sanitarium in Dallas, Texas. Dr. R. L. Spann, one of the city's outstanding surgeons, had been experimenting with several methods of treating cancer, none of them successful. I went to Dallas, talked with Dr. Spann, told him about the Hoxsey treatment, showed him a thick file of case histories and medical records. He immediately offered me a contract to join him in establishing a cancer clinic at his sanitarium.

The contract I signed was for a period of six months.

I'd already decided that if everything went well and conditions were favorable, at the end of that time I'd strike out on my own and in this booming city establish the greatest cancer clinic in the world.

I was heartily sick of being chased from city to city by the AMA. I was determined to continue treating cancer but I also wanted to settle down, raise a family, become a respected citizen in the community.

Ordeal by Fire

T HE Spann Sanitarium was a large, modern, two-story converted residence set far back on the lawn at a main intersection near the center of Dallas, with accommodations for some 30 bed patients. Here on March 9, 1936, we opened our cancer clinic.

Our first patient was Mrs. J. B. Whitehead of Wichita Falls, Texas. Hemorrhaging constantly from cancer of the cervix, 84 hours of radium had failed to relieve her condition. Her doctors had packed her in ice to stop the bleeding and told her family there was nothing more they could do for her. She was brought to us on a litter, so weak she couldn't stand on her feet.

After 33 days at the sanitarium on our treatment she was well enough to go home. She returned once a week. At the end of three months she had entirely recovered, the bleeding had stopped, she was discharged as cured.

Naturally members of her family were enthusiastic about her marvelous recovery, went out of their way to publicize it and recommend our treatment to other cancer victims. And quite naturally it wasn't long before the local medical society decided to step in and put a stop to such pernicious heresy. Doctors warned her husband—a car repair man on the railroad—that he must quit boosting the Hoxsey treatment or he'd lose his job. He told them to go to hell.

A few weeks later he was summarily fired. No reason whatsoever was given.

We immediately began action before the National Labor Relations Board to get his job back for him. The proceedings dragged on, necessitating numerous trips to Washington. In the meantime Whitehead, with a wife and seven others depending on him, was destitute. I arranged for the purchase of six washing machines and a 200-gallon hot water heater, and set him up in the laundry business.

Eventually the NLRB handed down a decision ordering the railroad to reinstate him on the job. Meanwhile the foreman of his department had died; by seniority rules Whitehead was entitled to that position. We forced the railroad to give it to him. When he was killed in an accident a few years later my wife and I took his son into our home and put the boy through college. He now is an instructor at a large Western university.

This was the first of many successful cases that demonstrated dramatically to cancer victims all over the Southwest what the Hoxsey treatment could do for them. And it showed them that we would go to bat for them if they got into trouble as the result of taking our treatment.

After six months of intensive work I decided I'd built up sufficient background and prestige in Texas to open my own clinic. Dr. C. M. Hartzog, M.D., who'd been assisting Dr. Spann, agreed to join me in the new venture. He had an excellent medical background. A graduate of the University of Tulane, he was licensed to practice in the States of Louisiana and Mississippi as well as Texas. We leased a small one-story building on the corner of

Bryan and Peak Street, remodelled it, and on December 5, 1936, began to treat patients there.

We took quarter-page ads in a suburban newspaper to announce our opening. About noon the first day the editor called me and told me that Dr. T. J. Crowe, secretary of the Texas State Board of Medical Examiners, had "suggested" he'd be wise to discontinue our advertising. We had a contract for 13 weekly insertions and I insisted that this commitment be honored. Somewhat reluctantly (and fearfully) the editor finally agreed.

Two days later Dr. Crowe himself showed up at the clinic. Pointing at the signs in our windows—"Bryan and Peak Cancer Clinic"—he demanded: "What do these mean?"

Dr. Hartzog calmly informed him that they meant just what they said; this was a cancer clinic.

Whereupon Dr. Crowe unleashed a 30-minute tirade. He told Hartzog that the latter wouldn't know a cancer if he saw one; he threatened Hartzog with loss of his license and jail; he swore he'd close our clinic if it was the last damn thing he ever did.

I grimly told him it *would* be the last thing he ever did, and ordered him off the premises.

The following day Dr. Hartzog was ordered to appear before the State Medical Board and show cause why his license should not be revoked. He quietly replied that he didn't intend to appear before the Board, nor would he sever his connections with the clinic. However he offered to appear before any impartial committee and prove to its satisfaction that we actually were curing cancer.

Needless to say, this offer was ignored.

At 9 A.M. on Dec. 22nd W. A. Rowan, an investigator for the State Medical Board, appeared at our clinic with warrants for the arrest of Dr. C. M. Hartzog, Harry M. Hoxsey and Mrs. Martha Hoxsey. The charge: practicing medicine without a license.

Dr. Hartzog protested that he was the only man in the clinic who treated patients, and produced his license to practice medicine in Texas. But Rowan brushed it aside, asserting that it had been cancelled the day before. I pleaded with them not to arrest my wife, who spent only two hours a day at the clinic installing a record system and never had anything to do with the treatment of patients, told him we had a six-months old infant at home who had to be nursed regularly. His brutal reply was:

"Any woman mixed up in a crooked racket like this should have sense enough to bring her baby up on a bottle!"

They wanted to put us in handcuffs and take us downtown on the street car! I refused to budge until we were permitted to go in my car, and they finally yielded. We were taken to the Dallas County Jail. It was four hours before we could contact my attorney and arrange bail. During this time Hartzog and I were confined in the bullpen with Federal prisoners, my wife in the women's section of the jail.

When the bail bonds finally were ready, and they brought Martha out, she was on the verge of collapse. She'd been locked up with a crew of prostitutes, dope addicts and other degenerate females. Obviously not one of them, she was subjected to all kinds of abuse and vile language. One of the women shoved a mop in her hands and ordered her to clean up the cell. When she refused, they ganged up on her, slapped her, knocked her down and kicked her.

It was all my attorney could do to restrain me from tearing the jail apart. I was ready to take anything the AMA could dish out, but not the humiliation and torture of an innocent woman. To this day I resent what they did to my wife more than any other outrage ever perpetrated against me or my family.

Trial was set for Jan. 4, 1937. We appeared on that date before Judge Winter King with a host of witnesses, ready and eager to have the case tried. The State requested an indefinite continuance, and over the protests of my attorneys it was granted. The very next day all three of us again were arrested on the same charge, signed by the same complainant. We again posted bond, and my attorneys obtained an injunction restraining the Medical Board from further arrests until the cases at issue had been tried.

While this case was still pending I was notified that four more warrants for my arrest on the same charge— practicing medicine without a license—had been issued by the district attorney of DeWitt County, in southern Texas. Now I'd never been in that county, much less practiced medicine there.

That same day I received a telephone call from Mrs. W. L. Jones of Yoakum, Texas, listed as the complaining witness in one of the new warrants. She told me that Dr. Crowe and Investigator Rowan had visited her home and urged her to sign the complaint against me. She informed them that she was dying of cancer of the intestines at the time she came to our clinic in Dallas for treat-

ment, indeed was so far gone that the doctor had advised
her husband to call in an undertaker! Now she was entirely
well, her weight had increased from 90 to nearly 180 lbs.,
our treatment had saved her life. So she'd refused to sign
the complaint.

Attorney Henry Smith, Dr. Hartzog and I immediately
drove to Yoakum. Through Mrs. Jones we contacted Tad
Moore, another "complaining witness" who'd refused to
sign the complaint to which his name was attached. They
accompanied us to Cuero, the county seat, and told their
stories to County Attorney Steve Hebert. When he
learned that the alleged offense had taken place in Dallas, and not in his county, he voided all four complaints.

Four weeks later Deputy Sheriff Bill Decker of Dallas
called me to ask what I was doing in LaVaca County
(adjoining DeWitt). It seemed that the prosecutor's
office there had just sent him three warrants for my arrest. The charge was the same: practicing medicine without a license. And the complaining witnesses were the
same as on the previous warrants!

Back we went to Yoakum, collected our two witnesses
and drove to Hallettsville, the county seat. Prosecuting
Attorney Walker listened attentively; when he heard
that the alleged witnesses didn't even live in his jurisdiction, he not only vacated the warrants but swore he'd slap
Crowe and Rowan in jail if they ever set foot in his office
again!

And so it went. During the three years 1937-39 more
than 100 separate charges of practicing medicine without a license were filed against me. Not a single one resulted in conviction. Each of them—including the original counts against Dr. Hartzog, my wife and myself—

eventually and after long delay were dismissed. Every time a warrant was issued it rated big headlines on the front pages of local newspapers. Dismissal of the charges invariably was buried in a few lines of fine print at the bottom of a back page of the same papers—if it appeared at all.

The AMA couldn't convict me or put me out of business. But by means of petty nuisance suits it could and did create a lot of unfavorable publicity for the clinic. And it kept me so wound up in legal tape that I actually spent more time in lawyers' offices and courtrooms than in the clinic! Similar tactics have forced more than one doctor to give up his fight against the AMA. But the only way to get me to quit was to lay me out in a coffin. And that was about all they *didn't* do to me.

About this time occurred one of the most incredible episodes in this entire fantastic history of persecution.

My principal foe in the Prosecutor's Office in Dallas was an assistant DA named Al Templeton. It was he who worked up most of the cases against me, and tried most of them in court. He had a younger brother, Mike, who lived with him.

Early in 1939 Mike Templeton developed cancer of the rectum. An operation was performed and the rectum removed, followed by a colostomy which short-circuited the colon and enabled him to discharge fecal matter into a rubber bag suspended at his side. In spite of this radical operation the cancer persisted and spread all over his body. He became an emaciated skeleton weighing only 83 lbs., kept alive by narcotics. The best specialists in the Southwest agreed he couldn't live much longer. When the odor of cancer became so strong that

Al's wife couldn't stand it any longer, their uncle, Lewis T. Carpenter, vice-president of the Southland Insurance Co. in Dallas, arranged to have the dying man removed to his home. A male nurse, Jack Howard, was hired to take care of him.

One day in the middle of November, Howard came to see me at the clinic. He said that Carpenter was anxious to explore any possibility of saving Mike's life. The doctors obviously couldn't do anything more for him. Would I try?

"Does Al know you're here?" I queried.

He shook his head. "No, we were afraid he wouldn't let me come if he knew."

"Okay, we'll do our best for him," I decided.

So Mike Templeton was brought to our clinic and started on the Hoxsey treatment. In two weeks he began to pick up weight. Within a month he abandoned narcotics. On Xmas morning he got out of bed, dressed, went over to Al's house and asked if he could borrow a shotgun.

"My God, you're not going to kill yourself?" Al exclaimed.

"No, I feel fine," was the reply. "I've gained 40 lbs. and I'm off the dope. I want to go rabbit hunting!"

His brother looked at him more closely. "You certainly look better. How in the world did you do it?"

Mike told him the whole story. Al was fit to be tied, but after chewing it over a couple of days he phoned me, said he wanted to see me.

"Fine," I replied. "Come right on over to the clinic."

He came, and we had a long talk. As he was leaving he asserted: "By God, after what you've done for my brother I'm not going to fight you any more. I'm resigning from the DA's office. They can get someone else to do their dirty work. You've got a case coming up soon, Harry. How'd you like me to represent you?"

I accepted with alacrity, and a few days later we walked into court together. When Dr. Crowe saw him at the defense table, he shouted:

"Wait a minute, Al. You can't represent this man. You prepared this case for the State!"

Al replied evenly: "I don't give a damn. Hoxsey saved my brother's life and I'll fight the whole State of Texas for him, if necessary."

Crowe and DA Andrew Patton put their heads together, went off to confer with the judge. The result was that all the charges against me prepared by Al Templeton were dropped. Those cases never did come up.

Mike got well, exhaustive examination by the same doctors who had once doomed him to death failed to disclose any signs of cancer. During the war he worked for the Government at Oak Ridge, Tenn. Always a heavy drinker, his death—some 10 years after discharge from my clinic—was attributed to acute alcoholism. Al Templeton later was elected County Judge. To this day we remain the best of friends.

The newspapers got hold of the Templeton story, and it created a terrific sensation. For once I had a favorable press. There was more sensation a few days later when Frank Ivey, another assistant DA, resigned and told newspapermen he was convinced that Hoxsey actually cured cancer. He too later defended me in Court.

I needed all the legal help I could get, for Dr. Crowe and his henchmen were closely following every move I made, hoping I'd put my head in a noose for them. Here is a letter he sent on Feb. 19, 1940, to Dr. George A. Gray, head of the local medical group at Sweetwater, Texas:

"This office desires to ascertain, if Dr. Carsie M. Hartzog and one Harry M. Hoxsey, who is not a Doctor and who operates a cancer clinic at Bryan and Peak Sts. in this city, are treating patients in your city for cancer. We are aware that they have made several trips to Sweetwater and we believe for the purpose of treating cancer.

"If you do not know of their activities in your community, kindly get in touch with your local physicians and associates and ascertain what they know about cancer cases being handled in Sweetwater. . . .

"If you learn anything of the activities of these men, please give us the names of persons treated and their addresses. If you find Dr. Hartzog is not registered in the District Clerk's office of your County, then we will proceed to file charges against both men for the illegal practice of Medicine.

"Keep this matter more or less under cover, except with your local associates, as we do not want this to get back to these parties. . . ."

Finally we obtained an injunction that put a temporary stop to the swearing out of phony warrants intended only to harass me, and to dissuade patients from coming to my clinic.

During the lull that followed I addressed numerous letters to the Dallas County Medical Society urging it to appoint a committee to investigate my treatment. All these letters were ignored. Finally I wrote Dr. W. W. Fowler, head of the Society:

"I cannot believe you will continue to ignore our request. I will bring a large number of persons who have been successfully treated at our clinic after radium, x-ray and surgery all have failed. These patients can tell their stories in their own way, the names of the doctors who treated them, operated upon them, gave them radium, x-ray, serum injections, blood transfusions and prescribed narcotics to be taken until death ended their misery.

"Doctor, let's forget about so-called ethics and meet this issue face to face. Let this treatment be compared by actual clinical tests where pathology, hospital records and all the data that can be gathered by your society will be used.

"We here at the clinic are constantly being condemned and harassed by organized medicine. Condemnation without opportunity to show our results before your association is wrong, unjust and unfair, and is locking the door of needless pain on mankind."

I offered to take 100 or more cases supplied by the Society, treat them free of charge under supervision of the Society and let the results speak for themselves.

There was no reply.

I sent out a form letter to every member of the County Medical Society urging them to arrange a meeting at which I might demonstrate our treatment. We mailed nearly 500 copies—and received exactly three replies. The remainder were too bigoted, or too fearful, to answer.

Then I wrote to Dr. Crowe:

"I cannot be led to believe that you and all the members of your association can turn your backs and close your eyes to facts and results that we are willing and eager to present to you. Dr. Crowe, in the name of suffering humanity use all your efforts and influence to bring about this meeting. Let's once and for all allow the facts about our clinic, whether good or bad, to be brought out into the open."

Again no reply. Instead, the AMA tightened its boycott against us.

One day in 1940 Dr. Marvin Bell, one of the pathologists who had been making biopsy reports for us, sent word that he wanted to talk with me. I drove down to his office in the Medical Arts Building.

"I'm sorry, Mr. Hoxsey, I'll have to quit doing pathologies for you," he said.

I asked why.

"Because the Medical Association told me I'd have to quit," was the reply. Within a week I got the same message from every pathologist in town who'd ever done business with us. We soon discovered that doctors, hospitals and laboratories all over the country had been warned not to send us any data relating to patients who came to us for treatment.

Meanwhile Crowe and his crew of hatchetmen were working day and night to round up witnesses who might be used to upset the injunction I had obtained, and send me to jail. The nature of their activities is revealed by the following confidential letter which later fell into my hands. It is typed on official stationery of the Texas State Board of Medical Examiners, dated Dec. 13, 1940, addressed to Jack W. Knight (Counsel for the Medical Board) in San Antonio, signed by W. F. McBride, State Board investigator in Dallas:

"After reading the attached copy of a report on a recent investigation you no doubt will think I have gone in for a lot of 'dusky' business. However, it seems that we are having a hard time connecting up a good case on Hoxsey where white people have been treated . . .

"I am sending you this for your comment and advice as to whether you think we could stand a chance to stick Hoxsey on evidence which is wholly testified to by negroes. It seems that these darkeys [sic] all have a clean record behind them and all have been questioned about any previous difficulty with the law and only one has ever been in court and paid a fine. This was Mamie Sneed who paid a one dollar fine in Corporation Court for running a red light on one occasion. . . .

"I have a few other clues and hope by Jan. 1st to be able to make a good case involving the treatment of some white person but if we are unable to do it, we would like to start working on him on this case if you think advisable.

"It seems that Dr. Crowe plans to have you come up here shortly after Jan. 1st and stay a few days, in order that you might go over all the evidence in cases involving Hoxsey and then file the best one or two. . . ."

They couldn't browbeat white people into testifying against me. And few reputable Negroes would do so, because they knew that this was about the only clinic in Texas where colored patients walked in the front door just like whites, got exactly the same treatment as whites, and more often than not were treated free of charge.

It took Dr. Crowe three months from the time this letter was written to prepare what he fondly hoped was a foolproof case against me.

One day in March 1941 Burt Whisnan, of the DA's office, walked into my clinic accompanied by two Dallas city detectives. He told me they had eight warrants for my arrest and were going to take me to jail. I asked why, since this was a county matter, the sheriff's office didn't make the arrest. Whisnan laughed and said:

"Old Crowe's been trying for some time to get you mugged and fingerprinted so's the FBI can check your record. He hasn't had much luck with the sheriff's office, so he turned the job over to us."

I put on my coat. "In that case, gentlemen, let's go. I have nothing to fear from the FBI."

My secretary phoned Al Templeton, and when we arrived at the city prison Al's wife was waiting for us with a writ of *habeas corpus*. The city had no jurisdiction over my case, it was a county matter. Hugh Hartson, chief of the Police Identification Bureau, advised me that I didn't have to submit to fingerprinting and photography. However I told him to go ahead; I was anxious to demonstrate that I did not have a criminal record.

So they sent my prints to Washington, and a few days later back came the reply that there was no record. Meanwhile I'd been transferred to County Jail and released on bond signed by Lewis T. Carpenter, my attorney's uncle. He said it was the least he could do to repay me for saving Mike.

Six times we appeared in court ready for trial. Each time we were accompanied by 125 to 150 patients clamoring to testify in my defense. Each time the State sought and received a postponement.

Finally on July 8th the trial started before Judge Winter King in Dallas County Criminal Court. Crowe, Knight and McBride had assembled 15 witnesses who testified that I had treated them or their relatives. Before they left the witness stand 6 of these turned hostile to the State and recanted their testimony, in whole or in part.

Throughout the trial Judge King's rulings consistently favored the prosecution and were prejudicial to the defense. The courtroom was crowded with cured patients who wished to testify in our behalf, but we were not permitted to put them on the witness stand. My wife was not allowed to testify. On one occasion, upholding a prosecution motion, the Judge stated that *"there is no evidence before the Court that Dr. C. M. Hartzog is a licensed physician"*—although such evidence had been presented. Over our objections, the Judge permitted Knight to present, in his closing argument to the jury, damaging material not brought out during the trial.

With the cards thus stacked against me, conviction was a foregone conclusion. Found guilty on five counts of practicing medicine without a license, I was fined $2,500 and sentenced to five months in jail—the stiffest penalty ever handed out in any medical practice suit.

We immediately appealed, listing no fewer than 50 reversible errors in the conduct of the trial.

While my appeal was pending, Crowe, determined to nail down the conviction, swore out a warrant for my arrest in Stephens County, Texas. The complaint stated that on three separate occasions I'd gone to Breckenridge and treated a local woman, Mrs. Sally Lane, and that she had died under my treatment.

Now it was true that Dr. Hartzog and I had treated Mrs. Lane for cancer of the womb and intestines after several doctors had given her up as hopeless. But the fact is she showed tremendous improvement under our treatment until she contracted influenza. She died of the flu, not of cancer.

In view of my previous conviction and appeal, the outcome of this case was extremely important to both sides.

Judge B. H. Atchison presided over this trial. The State presented four witnesses: the two sons, the daughter and son-in-law of the dead woman. It quickly developed that none of them held me responsible in any way for the death of Mrs. Lane. They testified that I'd never posed as a doctor, that Dr. Hartzog had examined and directed the treatment of the patient, that she'd shown remarkable improvement before coming down with the flu, and that we hadn't charged a penny for treating her. Although the State badgered and harried them mercilessly on the stand, they persisted in this testimony. The prosecution then rested its case—as thin a case as was ever presented in any courtroom.

Judge Atchison evidently thought so too. For after the noon recess, when my attorneys offered a motion for a directed verdict of not guilty on the grounds that the charges were not proven, he immediately granted it and instructed the jury to set me free.

A few months later, in April 1942, Crowe and his gang took another licking. Judge Hawkins, sitting on the bench in the Court of Criminal Appeals at Austin, found errors in my trial of the previous year. He reversed the conviction and ordered a new trial.

The State was in no hurry to try the case again, but my attorneys forced the issue. They went before Judge Joe B. Brown, who had just been elected to succeed Judge King, and demanded retrial or dismissal.

After hearing arguments on both sides, Judge Brown threw out the case against me. He said he didn't intend to let his court be used as an instrument of persecution, and directed the State Medical Board to cease molesting me until and unless it was prepared to present a *bona fide* case.

When a reporter asked Dr. Crowe why, in view of his assertion that I was a quack, the State couldn't get a single conviction against me that would stand up on appeal, he threw up his hands and declared: "This fellow

Hoxsey has been sued so many times and in so many States that he knows all the answers!"

Although my legal battles were far from ended, the favorable court decisions in 1942 marked a definite turning point in my 20-year battle with organized medicine. Our clinic was firmly established now, we'd legally won the right to treat cancer by unorthodox methods. I could now concentrate all my time and energy on improving the treatment and expanding our facilities and practice. Moreover World War II was in full swing now, the newspapers had little space to devote to the involved controversy between Harry M. Hoxsey and the AMA.

Of course the pressure continued. The State Medical Board filed suit to suspend or revoke Dr. Hartzog's license, harassed and threatened him so much that he finally had a nervous breakdown and was forced to leave the clinic. Dr. G. A. Hamlett, M.D. took his place. He too was continuously annoyed and threatened by Dr. Crowe until he finally resigned. Similar tactics have been employed against every doctor who has since joined the clinic.

Physicians outside the clinic who cooperated with us in any way, expressed approval of our treatment, or sent us patients were summoned before local medical boards and ordered to cease and desist, on penalty of losing their licenses. Many knuckled under; some fought their boards, and won.

One of the latter was Dr. Sam L. Scothorn, an outstanding osteopathic physician of Dallas (he is a former president of the American Osteopathic Association) whose wife at that time was under treatment at our clinic. On Oct. 17, 1947, Dr. Crowe sent him a letter or-

dering him to appear before the Board. Here is an
abridged copy of Dr. Scothorn's blistering reply.

"Inasmuch as it has been my privilege to serve on the
State Board under three different Governors, having served
with three different groups of doctors, I have learned that
usually doctors are honest and conscientious men. For that
reason I would like to respect your wishes and appear before
you.

"However I have learned that your reason for calling me
is because my wife was treated for cancer at the Hoxsey
Cancer Clinic, generally considered a quack institution. I
use "quack" purposely because since your Board was created
in 1907 the AMA has looked upon all irregulars as quacks.

"On the State Board . . . we have two groups—medical
and osteopathic—who claim to be highly ethical, yet surely
every one of you has heard that fee-splitting, abortions, and
narcotic violations are taking place through the activities
of some members of these highly-ethical groups. Yes, professional ethics are a sham, and the people know it.

"But because I decided not to let my wife be destroyed
by cancer and encouraged her to go to an irregular institution where she got beneficial treatment, I was told to give
up my time and go to the expense of appearing before your
Board and explaining my personal affairs.

"I have practiced in Dallas County for 39 years with
never a suit against me nor an insinuation of any kind
against my practice or character. I feel grossly insulted by
your letter and do not intend to appear before the Board
because, in my opinion, the letter smacks of conspiracy. . . .

He enclosed a detailed history of Mrs. Scothorn's case,
headed "HOW I LEARNED ABOUT THE HOXSEY
METHOD OF TREATING CANCER":

"My wife had both ovaries removed on May 4, 1944, and
diagnosis by biopsy was carcinoma of the left ovary. After
about 30 x-ray treatments during the next year she de-

veloped a severe pain in the liver area and nothing seemed to give her relief, she lost weight, her color was bad, she was nervous, sleepless and nauseated, so she went to another doctor who x-rayed her liver and found it enlarged and showing below the ileum bone. Her case seemed bad.

"On the 14th of July, 1945, Dr. Ira Drew of Philadelphia came into my office, stating he was in Dallas to see his son . . . and also visiting his old friend Harry M. Hoxsey, the cancer specialist. Of course he did not know that my wife had cancer or that I was like a drowning man reaching for a straw. I said, 'What do you know about him?' He replied, 'I know people living in Philadelphia today who were given up to die 15 years ago.'

"That same afternoon we went to the Hoxsey Cancer Clinic, and Mr. Hoxsey told me that he would treat 100 cases of cancer free of charge to prove the efficiency of his treatment, if we doctors would have the biopsies made so that we would be sure that he was treating cancer. He had previously made a similar offer to the Dallas County Medical Association . . .

"I told Mr. Hoxsey that my profession was perhaps as skeptical as the medical doctors, but I did get a few osteopathic physicians and we had 27 biopsies made. All 27 of these cases have been treated; all are still living except three; some of them were very bad breast cases.

RESULTS ON MRS. SCOTHORN

"After three months on the internal treatment her pain was gone, and her liver was reduced about 30 percent in size as shown by x-ray; she was x-rayed before and after taking the internal treatment. We think she definitely had cancer of the liver; however there was of course no biopsy made.

"For nearly a year after she had x-ray treatments her blood count was only 3 million reds; we were afraid she had too much x-ray. But after continuous osteopathic treatment, liver injections, Hoxsey's internal medicine and other accepted methods of treatment, her blood count reached 4.6 million for the reds recently.

"She has now lived three years and six months since she had surgery; her color is better; her pain is gone; she sleeps better; her liver is almost normal in size, and we think she is cured. If so, then the Hoxsey treatment did it, as we did nothing else after she discontinued the x-ray treatments . . .

"Strange to say, usually the ones who ridicule this treatment—doctors or laymen—are the ones too prejudiced and narrow-minded to go to the clinic and see for themselves the marvelous results that are often obtained."

Dr. Sam was just too much man for the Medical Board; it dropped the proceedings. He still practices medicine in Dallas. And his wife is still alive and in excellent health, and has had no recurrence of the disease in the intervening 8 years.

Even more heartless and cruel is the pressure exerted against patients at the clinic. They have been harassed and threatened by State Board investigators; they have even been refused emergency treatment by AMA doctors simply because they were taking the Hoxsey treatment!

Here is the story of one such patient, Mrs. E. S. Adams of Southgate, California, as set forth in a signed and notarized statement in our files:

"I became a patient at the Hoxsey Cancer Clinic for cancer of the breast on May 28, 1952.

"On or about February 18, 1953, I began to have very severe hemorrhages from my breast. I called the doctor in Southgate, California who had taken care of me before, to give me relief from this hemorrhage. He definitely refused to do anything for me because I was taking the Hoxsey treatment and said that if I would discontinue that and let him operate that he would try to help me.

"I also called another doctor from Long Beach, California who said that he was too busy to leave his office.

"Therefore it was necessary for me to take the plane and fly to the Hoxsey Cancer Clinic, Dallas, Texas, and get relief from severe hemorrhage. When I arrived there my clothing was saturated with blood and I was still bleeding very profusely. Bleeding was checked very easily within about 30 minutes after my arrival at the clinic."

Medical repression has been carried so far that even the relatives of Hoxsey patients are refused treatment by their own doctors. Recently we received an urgent telephone call from a man in Kansas. Suffering from a critical heart condition, he'd just had another attack. And his doctor refused to renew his prescription because his wife was undergoing treatment for cancer at the Hoxsey Clinic! *"Unless I get help I'll be dead within a few hours,"* he told us. One of our doctors immediately telephoned a prescription to the pharmacy nearest the man's home.

And these so-called doctors call us "unethical!" It is perfectly ethical to let human beings die for lack of medical attention; it is only unethical when you try to save lives!

However hard the AMA tried, it couldn't stop us from treating cancer, nor prevent hopeless cancer victims from flocking to our clinic. By the end of World War II the tiny building at Bryan and Peak no longer could accommodate our heavy patient load and the new equipment and laboratories necessary to carry on our work. Learning that Dr. Spann was about to retire, I arranged to purchase his sanitarium from him.

On June 1, 1946, we moved our clinic to the big building on Gaston Avenue, in Dallas. And that is where the Hoxsey Cancer Clinic now is located.

Two Senators and a State Legislature

W ITH the close of the war and the rapid expansion of the Hoxsey Clinic I decided to resume my fight for full recognition of the value of the Hoxsey treatment. Unable to persuade organized medicine to give us a hearing, we turned to the U.S. Government for help.

My first contact came about in October, 1945, through the help of my friend Charley Rodgers of New York. As a talent scout for USO shows during the war, Charley had occasion to meet many members of Congress. He took me to Washington and introduced me to some of his acquaintances on Capitol Hill. Among them were Reps. Virgil Chapman of Kentucky, Harold Earthman and J. Percy Priest, both of Tennessee.

They agreed that in view of the seriousness of the cancer problem Government intervention was warranted, and an official investigation of the Hoxsey treatment should be made. The proper Federal agency to conduct such an investigation, they informed me, was the National Cancer Institute, a bureau of the U.S. Public Health Service which spends about $20 million of the taxpayers' money each year for cancer research. They telephoned Dr. R. R. Spencer, Chief of the NCI, and arranged an appointment for me.

On October 19th, I appeared at the Public Health offices at Bethesda, Maryland, accompanied by the three

Congressmen and Charley Rodgers, who brought along a friend, Dr. H. H. Humphries, M.D. of Jacksonville, Florida. There were three other doctors in our party: Dr. Ira W. Drew, Dr. Sam Scothorn and Dr. Emil Platner. All of the latter had first-hand knowledge of numerous cases of cancer successfully treated by the Hoxsey method. In fact Dr. Scothorn's wife was then under treatment at our clinic.

We had a long talk with Dr. Spencer, and he promised that if I'd send him the records on 50 cases allegedly cured at my institution, with microscopic slides of biopsies proving that these patients actually had cancer when they began our treatment, we'd get an official investigation by his agency.

I returned to Dallas, put my secretary to work, and on Nov. 10th sent him the complete records on 60 cured cases. In a number of instances we were unable to provide biopsy slides because AMA doctors, hospitals and laboratories refused to furnish them to us. However each case was carefully documented with the names of doctors or institutions where these slides could be obtained.

While the NCI was studying these records Dr. Humphries paid a visit to our clinic. After remaining there a week and observing the treatment he sent the following telegram to Dr. Spencer:

"WHILE IN WASHINGTON ON OCTOBER 19TH I AC-CEPTED INVITATION OF CHARLES RODGERS TO AT-TEND PRELIMINARY MEETING IN YOUR OFFICE FOR OBSERVATION ONLY OF HOXSEY METHOD OF CANCER TREATMENT. THIS SO INTERESTED ME THAT I CAME TO DALLAS AT MY OWN EXPENSE TO MAKE PERSONAL INVESTIGATION. AFTER SPENDING THIS WEEK HERE I AM CLEARLY CON-

VINCED OF SUPERIORITY OF HOXSEY METHOD OVER RADIUM, X-RAY AND SURGERY AS I HAVE SEEN CURED CASES HERE WHERE ALL THREE HAVE FAILED. IN THE NAME OF HUMANITY I TRUST YOU WILL NOT DELAY BUT WILL GIVE YOUR DEEPEST SCIENTIFIC CONSIDERATION. EACH DAY'S DELAY PUTS THOUSANDS CLOSER TO THEIR GRAVES WHO COULD BE SAVED BY THIS METHOD. I HEARTILY ENDORSE AND RECOMMEND HOXSEY METHOD AS IT IS THE GREATEST BOON TO HUMANITY I HAVE SEEN DURING MY 42 YEARS PRACTICE AS PHYSICIAN AND SURGEON. I KNOW FAIR INVESTIGATION OF HIS PATIENTS AND RECORDS WILL VERIFY THIS.

H. H. HUMPHRIES, M.D.
JACKSONVILLE, FLORIDA

The NCI paid no attention to this or to numerous other communications from doctors who had witnessed the results of our treatment. Instead it immediately contacted the AMA. The impartiality of this Government agency's approach to the entire project may be judged by the following excerpt from its letter to Dr. Morris Fishbein:

"Mr. Hoxsey seems to have a persecution complex and states that he has been treated very unfairly by the AMA many years ago. He says you thought his remedy to be somewhat worthwhile and would have taken it up if he assigned over to you personally the entire rights."

Fishbein's reply can well be imagined.

Dr. Ralph R. Braund, Director of the USPHS Tumor Clinic, was assigned to check the records we had submitted. On Dec. 23, 1945, I received a copy of his report. An official communication summarized it as follows:

"Of the 40 cases of external cancer there was no histological biopsy proof of cancer in 25. And of the 20 alleged cases of internal cancer, no histological proof on cancer was submitted in 15.

"Obviously this does not meet the criteria laid down in the policy of our Advisory Cancer Council."

I was bitterly disappointed, disillusioned and shocked. Of course I had been aware all along that Dr. Spencer as well as his superior U.S. Surgeon General Thomas Parran were members of the AMA, as were nearly all the doctors associated with them. And thus amenable to AMA discipline. Nevertheless I'd sincerely believed that as Government employes they would conduct a full and impartial investigation, let the chips fall where they may.

The detailed report revealed that the case histories I'd sent them had not received the consideration and investigation they deserved. Let's take a look at that report.

It is broken down into two categories: external and internal cases. The 40 classified by the NCI as "externals" included skin, intraoral, urethra and breast cancer. Now in each of these cases there was unmistakable evidence of metastasis. And even medical students know that once cancer has metastasized it no longer can be considered merely an external lesion, it is an internal disease.

As to the lack of "histological biopsy proof," the report specifies:

"No histological report is available on the case of melanoma, though one might expect it was obtained since the lesion was removed surgically."

This refers to the case of Mrs. R. J. Hickman (see Chapter 18). I obtained a copy of the missing report; it is before me now. The analysis was performed by Dr. May Owen, M.D., at Terrell's Laboratories in Fort Worth.

The Pathological Opinion: "*Melanocarcinoma.*" If I could get it, why couldn't Dr. Braund?

The National Cancer Institute's report specifies:

> "We obtained the biopsy slide on the tongue lesion of Jesse A. Johnson. We fail to find cancer in it."

I have a copy of that biopsy report before me now, It too was made by Dr. Owen of Terrell's Laboratories. Pathological Opinion: *Squamous cell epithelioma, grade 2* (high 2). Dr. Owen called it cancer; Dr. J. C. Terrell, surgeon at the hospital in Stephenville, Texas called it cancer, and advised irradiation. Yet the NCI pathologist "failed to find" cancer!

The National Cancer Institute specifies:

> "There were three (3) breast lesions with positive biopsies. One of these, Mrs. O. G. Brown, was reviewed by Dr. Marvin Bell, the pathologist who made the original diagnosis of cancer. He states the slide shows only chronic inflammation."

I have before me a letter signed by Marvin D. Bell, M.D., and addressed to Dr. R. R. Braund, in which he states:

> "The slide which I find on Mrs. O. G. Brown shows chronic inflammatory tissues, and I do not know whether I was foolish enough to call this carcinoma at the time or if possibly I had another slide which did show carcinoma and was accidently discarded at the time."

There was no such uncertainty in Dr. Bell's mind six years before, when he made the original pathological diagnosis: "*Adenocarcinoma in the skin, recurrent, grade 2.*" It will be recalled that Dr. Bell got in trouble with the AMA in 1940 because he was doing biopsy analysis for our clinic. Could this explain his evasive reply in 1945?

As regards the cases admitted by the NCI as "internal" its report specifies:

> "In the case of Mrs. Lora Barnett, the Medicolegal Laboratory reports they have no record of any biopsy under that name, nor does their file of Dr. Dickens of Greenville, Texas, show any specimen submitted by him on or about August 5, 1949."

In fact the case history contained a photostatic copy of the biopsy report signed by V. G. Isvekov, M.D., LL.B., Director of the Medicolegal Laboratory at Houston, Texas. It was dated Aug. 5, 1939 (there was a typographical error in the report). The name of the patient is given as "*Mrs. Barnett,*" and it states that she was referred by *Dr. W. M. Dickens.*" Pathological conclusion: "*Adenocarcinoma of uterus*" (see Chapter 17).

The National Cancer Institute continues:

> "The case history of Mr. Frank Anderson leaves no doubt that there was extensive pulmonary pathology, though the nature of it is debatable."

The "debatable" pathology in this case was made at the world-famous Mayo Clinic, Rochester, Minn. by Dr. Broders, one of the most eminent pathologists in the country. Among the documents submitted was a letter signed by a doctor at the clinic (see Chapter 17) in which he stated that two doctors there had diagnosed cancer of the lung, that a specimen was removed and examined by Dr. Broders "who felt that the tissue was malignant." The only debatable feature in the case, it would seem, was how "a rather notorious cancer quack" could cure a lung cancer considered inoperable (and therefore incurable) by the greatest orthodox cancer clinic in the world!

It should be obvious by now that the NCI could have secured all the "histological proof" it needed if it had made a conscientious effort to do so. At the very least it had 20 biopsied "external" and internal cases of cancer where a cure was claimed. Surely that in itself was sufficient to establish that further investigation of the Hoxsey treatment was warranted. Obviously Dr. Spencer, Dr. Braund and company were not interested in seeking evidence to prove that an unorthodox cancer treatment was getting results in cases where orthodox medicine had failed. Nor, as we shall soon see, was their superior, the U.S. Surgeon-General.

The policy of the NCI, as regards cancer treatment, is identical with AMA policy. The proof is to be found in replies sent out on its stationery to various inquiries regarding the Hoxsey treatment. For example the following letter dated June 7, 1949, addressed to Mrs. V. J. McBride of Hoboken, N.J., and signed by Dr. R. F. Kaiser, Chief of the NCI Office of Technical Services:

"We have your letter asking advice on having your sister go to the Hoxsey Clinic. . . .

"Several years ago Mr. Hoxsey was asked to submit evidence to this Institute to prove his claim of a cancer cure. So far the records submitted to us by Mr. Hoxsey do not show that his claims are justified.

"Perhaps you do not know that the AMA has published several articles which label Mr. Hoxsey as a hoax and a charlatan. . . ."

Here is an official agency of the U.S. Government sending out, under Government franking privilege, AMA propaganda which the courts on two occasions (see the next chapter) held to be libelous and slanderous! It is a revealing indication of the AMA's decisive influence within administrative agencies of the Government.

Nevertheless I persisted in my efforts to promote Government intervention in the cancer controversy. The following year, with the help of another friend, I succeeded in persuading another member of Congress to conduct a personal investigation of the Hoxsey clinic.

U.S. Senator Elmer Thomas spent more than half his life in public service. A member of the Oklahoma State Senate from 1907 to 1920, he was elected to represent his State in Congress and after four years in the lower House won designation to the Senate. In more than 20 years of uninterrupted service in that Chamber he compiled an impressive record as an honest, conscientious and fearless legislator.

Shortly after the elections of 1946 one of his constituents—Tom R. Chapman, a well-to-do contractor of Lawton, Oklahoma—came to him with a strange and tragic story.

Early that same year Chapman's 12-year-old son Bobby had been stricken with cancer of the lymph glands. Nodes broke out all over the boy's body, many of them the size of hen's eggs; his neck became so swollen that it was thicker than his head. Local doctors were unable to stop the rapid advance of the disease, and on their advice the lad was taken to the Mayo Clinic. He was under x-ray treatment there for 7 weeks. Eventually doctors told the parents there was nothing more they could do, the boy was dying.

A friend of the family recommended the Hoxsey treatment, and the frantic father brought his son to us. After examination by my doctors I told Chapman: "I doubt that we can cure him, he's too far gone. But we're willing to try." We treated the boy for three weeks. During this time the nodes on his body were considerably reduced and his neck returned to normal size. Then Bobby developed pneumonia, one lung collapsed and on June 1st he died.

This was one case we did *not* cure. However the vast improvement in the boy's condition prior to death convinced the bereaved parents that we could have saved him, had he been brought to us earlier.

Two months after this tragedy the Chapman's noticed a small kernel under the knee of their remaining son, 3½-year-old Tommy. A week later there were nodes the size of a man's thumb on his neck, groin, arms and spleen. Their worst fears confirmed by medical opinion, without further ado the parents brought us the child and we put him under treatment.

In four days the nodes stopped growing. Two months later they disappeared. At the end of six months Tommy was discharged as cured. There has been no recurrence of cancer; today the boy is a normal, healthy child.

His son's life spared, Chapman decided he owed a duty to other cancer sufferers. He got in touch with the Oklahoma Medical Society and offered to arrange for treatment—under the Society's supervision—of 25 patients at the Hoxsey Clinic.

His offer was rejected.

He addressed the same offer to the American Cancer Society, with the same result.

Then he got in touch with Sen. Thomas. "Cancer is a

national tragedy," he told the Senator. "If there is a cure for it, you and I should know about it, and the American people should hear about it."

The Senator agreed. But he refused to believe that organized medicine would not investigate any cure for cancer, however fantastic. Doctors and hospital authorities whom he consulted advised him it was *"a waste of time"* to concern himself with *"that quack Hoxsey."* However at Chapman's insistence he agreed to talk with a dozen or more constituents in and around Lawton who had taken or were then taking the Hoxsey treatment. And from them he got tales of fabulous and almost unbelievable cures. His curiosity and sense of duty aroused, he promised to visit our clinic at the earliest opportunity and see for himself.

Soon thereafter a group of 15 osteopaths from various sections of the country came to the Hoxsey Clinic to study our treatment. We sent a wire to the Senator suggesting that this would be a good time to pay us a visit. He arrived in Dallas on Feb. 2, 1947.

We showed him through the clinic, opened all our records to him, brought in about 125 patients and former patients to present first-hand testimony as to their experiences with the Hoxsey treatment. The Senator picked cases out at random, mostly patients from Oklahoma and Texas. When he'd questioned about 27 of these, with the acceptance of visiting doctors, he said he'd seen and heard enough. In an interview with AP, UP, newspaper and magazine reporters who attended the hearing, he declared:

"I'm not a doctor, don't know cancer when I see it. However I feel that I have gone into the matter sufficiently to justify asking medical authorities to investigate further. If this is a real cure for cancer, as evidenced by testimony here today, then it should at least be given a fair test and made available to the world. If not, the man must be exposed."

I agreed, and issued a challenge in which I offered to take 100 ex-servicemen with pathologically-proven cancer and treat them free of charge. If I failed to cure 80 percent of the cases we treated, I promised to close my clinic and stop treating cancer.

On his return to Washington Sen. Thomas wrote Surgeon-General Parran and urged him to investigate the Hoxsey method. In reply he received the following:

"At my request Dr. Spencer had a copy of a recent statement appearing in the *Journal of the AMA* forwarded to your office. This statement contains so much factual and incontrovertible evidence concerning the Hoxsey Cancer Clinic that I would hesitate to spend public funds on a project such as this."

To allay the Surgeon-General's commendable concern about spending public funds I wrote to him and offered to pay all the expenses of any official investigation of my method. I offered to produce conclusive evidence that the "factual and incontrovertible evidence" he referred to was nothing but a fabrication of lies.

There was no reply.

Sen. Thomas spent four months begging public and private authorities for an investigation of the Hoxsey Clinic. Finally on June 2, 1947, he wrote me:

"It seems that the medical fraternity is highly organized and that they have decided to crush you and your institution, if at all possible. I have had a few 'rounds' with the heads of all the medical organizations as well as the Public Health Service here in Washington, and it seems that the public officials are afraid that if they make any move, or say anything antagonistic to the wishes of the medical organization, that they will be pounced upon and destroyed. In other words, the public officials seem to be afraid of their jobs and even of their lives. This represents a most serious case and I am at a loss to know how to proceed.

"I am of the opinion that what the medical organization does will be repeated by the several state organizations in the event any Congressman or Senator starts out to publicly oppose their program. I have done what I could to have your remedy, or at least the record of your accomplishments, considered and passed upon but, to date, the authorities here have refused to act. . . ."

Here was a sorry state of affairs, a medical dictatorship that dominated even the organs of Government. We had just overthrown Fascist tyranny in Europe; yet we were helpless and forced to bow to the tyranny of a small clique of medico-politicos in our own land! With more than 200,000 Americans dying of cancer every year, the Government couldn't find out whether all or some of them could be saved by our treatment!

Sen. Thomas soon discovered that the fears of public officials were not unfounded. When he came up for re-election the AMA and the Medical Society of his State campaigned vigorously against him, and he was defeated. He now conducts a private law practice in Washington, D.C.

Recently, in reply to an inquiry from a national magazine, he issued the following statement:

"I still get many letters from people in various states asking my opinion of the Hoxsey method. My answer to all of them is the same; if I had cancer I would try the Hoxsey method; if any member of my family or any friend had it, I certainly would recommend that they try that method.

"That's a pretty good indication how I feel about this treatment."

About the same time Sen. Thomas first began his investigation two members of the Oklahoma State Legislature—Rep. Charles Ozman and Sen. Homer Paul—became interested in accounts they heard of the Hoxsey treatment. Learning that more than 150 citizens of their State were then taking the treatment they introduced a resolution for a joint legislative investigation of the Hoxsey Clinic.

In debate on the measure Sen. Paul charged that Dr. Morris Fishbein, editor of the AMA *Journal,* was chiefly responsible for blocking investigation of our method. Dr. Louis Ritzhaupt, the only medical man in the State Senate, replied that Dr. Fishbein *"no longer controls"* the AMA, and that he was sure the medical profession in this State was *"perfectly willing"* to investigate thoroughly any treatment for cancer.

The Oklahoma State Medical Society and the AMA soon demonstrated that Dr. Ritzhaupt was talking through his hat. They deluged every member of the Legislature with telegrams and reprints of AMA editorials attacking me and my father; they fought tooth and nail to prevent the investigation.

Despite determined outside opposition the resolution was approved overwhelmingly in both Houses and a joint investigating committee was named. It consisted of five Senators (Homer Paul, Bill Goody, M. O. Counts, H. B. Binns, Arthur L. Price) and five Representatives (Charles Ozman, Dr. A. E. Henning, Jack Coleman,

Owen Summers, W. A. Burton, Jr.). This Committee appointed three medical advisors: Dr. Grady Matthews, State Health Commissioner; Dr. Reynold Patzer, Professor of Surgery at the University of Oklahoma; Dr. Howard C. Hopper, Professor of Pathology at the same institution. All of them were good AMA members.

The AMA *Journal* editorially attacked the Oklahoma State Legislature for daring to investigate Hoxsey.

The committee arrived in Dallas on the evening of March 11, 1947. The hearing was scheduled to begin the following morning at 9 A.M. However, at that hour only 9 legislators showed up. Dr. Henning and his three medical colleagues were closeted with officials of the Dallas County Medical Society. It was nearly 10 o'clock before they made their appearance at the clinic.

In six hours the investigators heard more than a score of patients and ex-patients testify under oath that they were cured of cancer by the Hoxsey treatment. Dr. Patzer assisted in bringing out the pertinent medical facts. At the conclusion of the testimony I was asked to present records to document the testimony and prove beyond doubt that we cure internal cancer. I promised to do so.

The three medical advisers agreed to return that evening and help me select the proper documentation. But they never showed up!

At the request of Sen. Paul, presiding officer of the Committee, I then went through my files, selected 60 cases of internal cancer successfully treated at the clinic, completely documented them with case histories, pathological reports, x-ray and other photos, and personally delivered them to the Committee. These were all turned over to Dr. Patzer so that he and his colleagues could study them and hand in a report as to their opinion of the evidence we'd offered.

Several weeks having passed without further development, I drove to Oklahoma City and dropped in to see Rep. Ozman. In my presence he telephoned Dr. Patzer, who informed him that the matter had been submitted to the AMA and a complete report would be forthcoming within a few days.

A week later I returned to Oklahoma City. This time I went to see Sen. Paul. He telephoned Dr. Patzer, requested him to come to his office. When the doctor arrived we asked him what had happened to the report on the 60 cases I'd submitted. Dr. Patzer assured us that they were under study, and the report would be ready soon.

A carefully-worded three-page medical report finally was presented to the Senate. It stated that my refusal to divulge the ingredients of our medicines *"makes it impossible to evaluate its possible effect."* It shrugged off the 60 case histories I'd submitted as *"insufficient"* for a verdict as to whether we cure cancer. And it concluded:

"It is our opinion that Mr. Hoxsey has not demonstrated effectiveness of his 'internal medicine' in treating internal cancer. His experimental studies strongly indicate that the medication which he advocates has no beneficial effect upon cancer and that, furthermore, it is toxic."

In an angry, 30-minute speech on the floor of the Senate a few days later (April 15) Sen. Paul vigorously contradicted every particular in the medical report. He declared that any investigation into the Hoxsey treatment would be "hampered, browbeaten and threatened" by the AMA:

"It would do no good whatsoever to file a written report on this investigation. We can never get any cooperation on this Dallas cure from the American Medical Association—and I might as well say the Oklahoma Medical Association too.

"These doctors who went with us down there stayed through the meeting with fear and trembling in their hearts. We tried to get them to help us make out a report two weeks ago but they wouldn't do it until they had contacted the AMA to find out what to do.

"We actually took testimony from 35 or 36 patients, and the testimony we received proved in my mind that these people—regardless of their cancer condition before treatment—were completely cured."

As to the 60 case histories we'd submitted:

"The doctors said they couldn't go by these files because they had been unable to make a personal examination on the patients. I know why they say that. They're afraid of having their licenses revoked!"

And there was nothing the sovereign State of Oklahoma could do to correct this scandalous situation!

There is a sardonic postscript to this episode. Since then one of the doctors who said we'd failed to demonstrate the effectiveness of our treatment has secretly sent us several cancer patients. He is merely one of a growing number of physicians—all of them staunch members of the AMA—who "bootleg" patients to us, first making them promise they will never reveal the source of the recommendation.

As Sen. Paul stated, they're afraid they'll be thrown out

of the Association and their licenses revoked if their heresy is discovered!

In 1951 another member of the U.S. Congress, Sen. William Langer (of North Dakota) paid a visit to the Hoxsey Clinic, examined our records and heard the testimony of numerous patients. On his return to Washington he sponsored a resolution (S. Res. 142) directing the Committee on Labor and Public Welfare to conduct a full-dress investigation to determine whether *"methods employed by the Hoxsey Cancer Clinic of Dallas, Texas in the treatment of cancer have proved a cure for the same disease."*

Naturally this aroused the furious opposition of the AMA. In an effort to enlist as wide support as possible among other members of Congress, Sen. Langer then substituted another resolution (S. Res. 186) directing the above committee to make *"a full and complete study and investigation of the efficacy of methods used in the treatment of cancer in any hospital or clinic which has been in operation for at least ten years and which presents pathological proof of cures of internal cancer in at least five cases."*

The AMA succeeded in getting this resolution bottled up; it never was reported out of committee. Most Congressmen vividly remembered the AMA purge the previous year (see Chapter 8) and didn't hanker for another dose of the same medicine.

Suits for Slander

As MIGHT BE EXPECTED, the AMA did not content itself with passive resistance to my persistent efforts to obtain a Government investigation. Regardless of its outcome such an investigation would set a dangerous precedent for further Government intervention in medical affairs. I had become a serious threat to the prestige, authority and privileges of the medico-politicians who dominate the healing profession in this country.

The alarm was sounded in a 3½-column lead editorial of the AMA *Journal* (March 15, 1947) headed "HOX-SEY—CANCER CHARLATAN." For the most part a reprint of old slanders previously published in the same paper about me and my father, the editorial wound up:

"Apparently Harry Hoxsey in his performance in Dallas, Texas, is being aided by osteopaths, who are licensed to practice medicine in that state. Apparently he has been successful in hoodwinking and deceiving eminent jurists and other important persons to the extent that they have given him tacit if not actual support. Apparently his performances and his success have caused him to believe that it is now possible for him to exploit widely his method of treating cancer and that he can get away with it!

"How long will the complacent authorities of such states as Texas continue to tolerate Harry M. Hoxsey?"

In response to this goad the Texas State Medical Board

girt up its loins and made another desperate effort to close down my clinic by fair means or foul.

A new warrant on the old charge of practicing medicine without a license was sworn out against me. This time I was accused of personally performing an operation upon the breast of one of our patients, Mrs. A. M. Richards of Fort Worth, Texas. It was alleged that she died as the result of our treatment. To make the charge more binding, a few weeks later the husband of the deceased filed a $75,000 damage suit against me.

As in previous instances, this complaint was completely false.

Mrs. Richards came to us for treatment in August, 1945. She was suffering from cancer of the breast which had metastasized under the arm, to the back and neck. After several months of treatment all the cancer masses had cleared up except a small nodule under her arm, and it was reduced to about half its original size.

In July 1946 the patient and her husband announced that they had decided to have the remaining nodule removed surgically. Dr. Durkee, then Chief of Staff at our clinic, recommended that they consult Dr. Harry Taylor, an osteopathic surgeon who owned a hospital at Lewisville, Texas. They went there, and the operation was performed on July 17th. After the operation Mrs. Richards took a series of intensive x-ray treatments. On June 25, 1947—nearly a year after she'd abandoned the Hoxsey treatment—the unfortunate woman died.

These basic facts were concurred in by both sides at the trial which opened in Dallas County Court before Judge Herbert Marshal on Jan. 12, 1948. The prosecution contended that I had personally treated Mrs. Richards at the clinic and personally performed the operation on her in the hospital at Lewisville. And that she might still be alive if she'd gone to an authorized hospital for treatment, instead of the Hoxsey Clinic. We denied all three charges.

If there was any doubt who inspired this suit, it was thoroughly cleared up by the husband of the deceased when he took the witness stand. Richards admitted that Lloyd Rhode, an investigator for the State Medical Board and George Frentzos, an investigator for the District Attorney's office, had visited him several times shortly after the death of his wife and persuaded him to sue me.

The prosecution put on a number of doctors who testified that, from the *"description"* of the symptoms (!), surgery performed at the time Mrs. Richards first came to our clinic "might have cured" her.

It also put on the stand two disgruntled ex-employees of the clinic. They testified that they saw me administer treatment to Mrs. Richards as well as other patients, and at various times perform minor operations on patients *"with a razor blade."* One of these witnesses was a doctor who had been discharged (for drunkenness) by me, and we put in evidence a threatening letter he'd written after he was fired, trying to shake me down for $300 per month for 5 years. The other was a former head nurse who had taken leave of absence from her job; she'd resigned when we refused to reinstate her in her old position.

Then the State pulled a trump card out of its sleeve. It put on a surprise witness who identified herself as Constance Brown, a registered nurse for 23 years. She testified that she frequently had called for patients at the

Hoxsey Clinic, at which time she had seen and talked with me, and made the acquaintance of Mrs. Richards. On July 17, 1946, she was nursing a private patient at Dr. Taylor's hospital and happened to walk into the operating room. She swore that I was there, and that she saw me perform the operation on Mrs. Richards.

Both Dr. Taylor and I stared at her in amazement. Neither of us had ever seen her before!

In my defense, clinic employees testified that I myself had never treated any of our patients, nor operated on them with razor blades. They said they'd never seen Constance Brown at our establishment. Dr. Taylor testified that it was he who actually performed the operation on Mrs. Richards. Both he and his wife (who assisted in the operating room) swore they'd never seen Mrs. Brown in their hospital and that I was not in the operating room or anywhere else on the premises on the day of the operation.

This trial ended in a stalemate. Faced with such sharply contradictory testimony, the jury finally gave up and announced that it was unable to reach a verdict.

We immediately put investigators on the trail of the mysterious Constance Brown, and they discovered a number of interesting things. For one thing, she was not a registered nurse as she had testified, but a practical nurse. Her patients said that she was a *"very inefficient nurse,"* and *"very unreliable with the truth."* We discovered that she could not have been at our clinic at the time she claimed, because the dates did not correspond with those on which her patients had appeared for treatment. Even more important, the patient she allegedly nursed at Dr. Taylor's hospital—a Mrs. Paul

Johnson—said she was not in that hospital on the date of the operation, and didn't even know Mrs. Brown, much less employ her as a nurse!

The $75,000 civil damage suit brought against me by Richards was tried four months later before Judge W. L. Thornton in Dallas County Court. The plaintiff charged that my negligence contributed to the death of his wife. Said negligence consisted in administering the Hoxsey treatment and performing an operation for which I was not qualified.

The witnesses on both sides were substantially the same as in the previous contest. But this time when Constance Brown took the stand we were prepared for her: my attorneys tore her testimony apart, we put on rebuttal witnesses, and she was thoroughly discredited. In addition, 41 former patients took the stand and testified that we'd cured them of cancer.

The hearing lasted almost three weeks. At its close Judge Thornton handed the jury 23 issues to determine. On June 4th after 8 hours of deliberation, the jury returned a verdict resolving all 23 issues in my favor. It ruled:

That the treatment Hoxsey gave Mrs. Richards did not constitute negligence;

That Hoxsey did not advise the operation performed upon her at Dr. Taylor's hospital;

That Hoxsey did not perform this operation;

That Mrs. Richards died from causes other than negligence on Hoxsey's part;

That her abandonment of the Hoxsey treatment was the approximate cause of her death;

That she died of cancer treated in the manner approved by the AMA.

In an unexpected burst of enthusiasm one Texas daily headlined its story "JURY FINDS CANCER CURE DE-VELOPED." And Judge Thornton, asked by newspaper-men to comment on the verdict, declared that in his opinion this was "the most important case in the last 100 years."

We then went before the Grand Jury, turned over the evidence we'd uncovered and demanded that Mrs. Brown be indicted for perjury. But there was no indict-ment. The State obviously did not wish to publicize the fact that I'd been framed on phony testimony.

Significantly enough, no attempt was ever made to re-try the criminal case against me, and the charge even-tually was dismissed.

Even before this battle was over, a much bigger one was shaping up. For between the two trials in the Rich-ards case the AMA had succeeded in getting a vicious attack upon me printed in the largest chain of newspa-pers in the nation.

The article, entitled "BLOOD MONEY," appeared in the Feb. 15, 1949, issue of the *American Weekly,* the Sun-day magazine supplement of the Hearst Publications. It was published in 20 newspapers with a combined circu-lation of nearly 9½ million copies and read by an esti-mated 20 million people. The story carried a double by-line: "by Morris Fishbein, M.D., Editor, *Journal of the American Medical Assn.,* and William Engle" (a Hearst feature writer). It was part of a series on so-called "Medi-cal Hucksters."

The format of the piece was typical of the lowest kind of yellow journalism. Most of the double spread was taken up by a lurid drawing in color of a poor woman on her couch of pain surrounded by sorrowing children and a mournful dog. She was handing over her last few dollars to a leering caricature of a quack decked out in swallow-tail coat, razor-sharp trousers, fancy scarf with a big diamond stickpin and white spats.

The text was slanted to appeal to the emotions of the reader, rather than his logic. It began:

"All the other wicked medical fakes, firing hope and darkening it to despair, pale beside the savagery of the cancer charlatans. They look like men, they speak like men, but in them, pervading them, resides a quality so malevolent that it sets them apart from others of the human race. . . .

"They slay their patients as guiltily as if they knifed them in the heart, and they stay within the letter of the law."

A few more paragraphs of rabble-rousing purple prose, and the writers got down to naming names:

"Among today's cancer 'healers,' the AMA charges, a former coal miner is boldest, has the largest following and even has engaged the interest of some prominent men. He is Harry M. Hoxsey, who inherited a 'cancer cure' from his father, a dabbler in veterinary medicine, faith healing and 'cancer curing,' who, himself, died of cancer."

The distinguished author had inherited from his spiritual father the technique of the big lie: "*Make up a lie that's big enough, repeat it often enough and people will believe it!*" Adolf Hitler was dead, but the Hitler of American medicine ranted on.

The rest of the article warmed over the same old tripe about me and my treatment previously dished out in the columns of the AMA *Journal*. Indeed entire paragraphs had been lifted, word by word, from Fishbein's editorials. He complained again that I was "*hoodwink-*

ing and deceiving eminent jurists and other important persons" into giving me their support. Again he used the big lie to explain away living evidence that the Hoxsey treatment cures cancer:

"Mountebanks claim cures and bring support of those who believe they have been cured, when the diagnosis has never been made by scientific methods."

How scientific can you get? We had biopsy reports from AMA pathologists and institutions; we had case histories from AMA hospitals and clinics; in nearly all cases the original diagnosis was made by an AMA doctor; we had microscopic slides of cancerous tissue taken from our patients; we had x-ray negatives and photographs displaying visible proof of cancer.

With unmitigated gall the writers added:

"Hoxsey has had more than 20 years in which to prove such virtues as might have existed in his method. Such proof has never been forthcoming."

Not a whisper about the scores of letters I'd written over the years to Fishbein and other AMA officials, begging for an opportunity to give them the proof he now said was *"not forthcoming."* Nary a word about the AMA's repeated refusal to investigate, and its stubborn opposition to investigation by Federal and State agencies. No mention whatsoever of the hundreds of patients who'd testified in open court that we'd cured them of cancer.

In short this was a typical AMA fabrication of misstatements and outright lies. Not a scintilla of evidence, scientific or otherwise, accompanied the charges. Diarrhea of words, constipation of proof. The AMA ordered hundreds of thousands of reprints and shipped them to doctors, public officials and laymen all over the country!

There's a peculiar story behind this article and the circumstances surrounding its publication.

Early in 1946 while I was in New York on business my friend Sigmund Janis (then head of the Colonial Airlines) introduced me to the city editor of the New York *Journal and American,* one of the leading Hearst newspapers. The editor, Paul Schoenstein, was highly skeptical about my treatment, but said he'd send a reporter to interview me. I met the reporter, William McCullam, the next day. He too was frankly cynical, so I invited him to our clinic to see for himself. He said he'd discuss the proposition with Schoenstein.

I returned to Dallas. A few weeks later—about May 4th—McCullam walked into my office at the clinic. With him was a Dr. Lucas, a prominent New York specialist. McCullam told me bluntly:

"Hoxsey, I've been sent down here to investigate you and your treatment. If you're a quack, we're going to expose you. But if you really cure cancer, we'll put your story before the public and see that you get an investigation by some authoritative medical group."

That suited me fine. "I don't care what you print about me as long as you tell the truth," I declared. "Let your conscience be your guide." I gave them free run of the clinic, instructed my staff to cooperate with them 100 percent.

McCullam and Lucas spent a week in the clinic. They quizzed doctors and nurses, donned white coats to supervise the treatment of patients, eventually interviewed about 400 cases in various stages of treatment.

They ransacked my files, waded through thousands of case histories, volumes of court testimony, stacks of photos and x-ray negatives. They talked with my foes as well as my friends, interviewed Dr. Crowe of the State Medical Board, local AMA officials, scores of pathologists and other doctors.

At the end of that time we had a meeting in my office to hear their verdict. Sigmund Janis was there, he'd flown down in his private plane. And Dr. Lucas said, in substance:

"There's no question in my mind that the Hoxsey treatment benefits some types of cancer. Whether it benefits all types, I am unable to say at this time. It definitely merits further investigation."

I was elated. Guarded as this oral opinion was, I felt it would carry weight with the Hearst editors and they would start the ball rolling for an AMA investigation.

Dr. Lucas and McCullam went out together. When they were alone the reporter asked him: "Now that you've come to the conclusion that the Hoxsey treatment definitely benefits some types of cancer, what are you going to do about it?"

"Nothing!" the physician replied.

McCullam was incredulous. "You mean to say you are convinced this man's treatment helps cancer victims, and you won't tell anybody about it?"

The elderly doctor smiled. "Look, son," he said quietly. "When you're as old as I am, you'll realize that discretion is the better part of valor."

He left the following morning; I never saw him again. But McCullam came back and reported the conversation. He was deeply disturbed. "Harry, I'm convinced you're curing cancer," he declared. "But I'm taking on a hell of a responsibility if I put that in print. I've got to be sure I'm right. I'd like to stay here another week and go over your material with a fine-tooth comb."

"You can stay here as long as you like," I assured him.

McCullam continued his investigation. At the end of the second week, as he was about to return to New York, he told me:

"I'm going home and write the truth as I see it. And I'm going to do everything in my power to get you an AMA investigation. If I didn't, I'd have the lives of thousands of cancer victims on my conscience."

He was as good as his word. On his return he wrote a series of six articles objectively stating the facts turned up by his examination. He stated clearly that he was no doctor, and therefore was not qualified to determine whether Hoxsey actually cured cancer. But he'd seen enough to reach the conclusion that the Hoxsey treatment warranted a full-fledged medical investigation. His articles were documented with photos and photostatic copies of medical records, biopsy reports and correspondence. To these he attached a notarized letter from me, as follows:

"I, Harry M. Hoxsey of Dallas, Texas do hereby challenge the U.S. Government, any recognized medical association, or any medical institution to supervise my treatment of 100 cases of cancer. Each case, to be selected by me, must be attested first by the U.S. Government pathology as cancer.

"I guarantee cures in over 80 percent of the 100 cancer cases within 12 weeks by use of my method and further guarantee no recurrence of the disease for five years in each cured case.

"I further challenge any recognized physician in the world to duplicate this statement."

McCullam turned the completed material over to Schoenstein, who read it carefully. The editor sat on it for days, worrying and fretting about it. He could find nothing wrong with the articles except that they were too hot to handle. So he passed them on to the front office. "Let them make the decision," he told his reporter.

Weeks went by, and the articles didn't appear. One day I received a phone call from McCullam. He was so mad he could scarcely speak.

"They've turned the articles down, Harry. They've checked with the AMA, it has convinced them that your treatment is worthless and you are a quack. I'm sorry, it's no use arguing with them. I'm still convinced you're curing cancer, and I'll do what I can to help you. If there are any new developments, let me know."

At the beginning of 1947, when U.S. Sen. Thomas was due in Dallas, I invited McCullam to sit in on the hearing. He flew down, joined in questioning some of the witnesses, and took a transcript of the proceedings home with him. Still the Hearst papers did not publish his articles.

One year later, the article "BLOOD MONEY" appeared in the Sunday supplement of the New York *Journal and American,* and 19 other newspapers across the country. Subsequently we learned why the "front office" turned down the favorable report of its own investigator and published instead the scurrilous piece by the AMA official.

McCullam's articles had been sent to the Hearst sci-

ence editor, Gobhind Behari Lal, and the latter brought
them to Fishbein's attention. Reading them, my arch-
enemy hit the ceiling. The reporter had been taken in by
a notorious quack, he asserted. If the Hearst papers
wanted to render a real public service they would cooperate with the AMA in exposing frauds like the Hoxsey
treatment.

It was unnecessary to mention the fact that the AMA
indirectly controls millions of dollars worth of advertising—everything from tooth paste and aspirin to cigarettes and ladies' girdles.

Nearly 2,000 years ago Pontius Pilate, confronted by
the great Healer, cynically observed: "What is truth?"
The Hearst organization piously washed its hands, and
instead of taking its own investigator's word assigned
William Engle to collaborate with Dr. Fishbein on a
series of articles exposing "medical quackery."

And that's the background for "BLOOD MONEY."

I promptly entered civil suit for libel against Morris
Fishbein, William Engle, W. R. Hearst, Jr., the *American
Weekly*, Hearst Consolidated Publications Inc., and the
AMA. The suit was filed at 9 A.M., and promptly reported
on the radio. Within two hours the Texas State Medical
Board rushed down and filed against me 16 separate and
distinct charges of practicing medicine without a license!
It was purely a propaganda move, designed to steal newspaper headlines and distract public attention from my
suit against Fishbein and Hearst. Every one of these
charges was dropped as soon as they'd served their purpose; they were never brought to trial.

Fishbein, Hearst, Engle and the AMA refused to accept our summonses. Since they resided and maintained

headquarters outside the jurisdiction of the Court, there was no way to compel them. We were forced to drop them from the roster of defendants. However the libelous article had appeared in a Hearst paper in Texas, the San Antonio *Light,* so the Hearst Publications had to defend the action.

My friends tried to dissuade me from going through with it. I had trouble enough battling the AMA, they argued; now I was taking on a rich and powerful journalistic empire with representatives in every major city in the country and every capital on the globe. They'd bring in the best legal and medical talent in the country against me. It was pitiful, they'd murder me in court!

I reminded them that the fight was not of my choosing. Nobody, however rich or powerful, was going to push me around with impunity. I had to put an end to these slanderous attacks not only for the sake of my reputation and that of my family, but for the sake of millions of people all over the world who had a vital stake in this controversy.

The hearings opened March 16, 1949, in the U.S. District Court in Dallas. On the bench was Judge William H. Atwell, one of the most learned and respected jurists in the Southwest. The trial lasted three full days, including two night sessions, during which time the testimony of some 75 witnesses was heard and a record of close to 2,000 pages compiled.

With the defendants pleading justification, the central issue became the effectiveness of the Hoxsey treatment. Our first witness was Dr. J. B. Durkee, at that time Medical Director of the clinic. He analyzed the scientific background of the treatment, described its application

in more than 5,000 cases he personally had examined
and treated. A most convincing witness, he stood up well
under cross-examination.

When we called our first cured patient to the stand,
defense counsel objected strenuously. They maintained
that persons without medical training are incompetent
to testify whether they have or at one time had cancer.
The elderly judge overruled them. He referred them to
the Good Book, to the story of the two blind beggars at
the Temple cured by Peter and John:

"They testified before the people: '*All we know is, we
were blind and now we see.*' Certainly, gentlemen, they
were competent witnesses to that fact."

Altogether we put 57 competent witnesses to the fact
that we cure cancer on the witness stand. They cited the
names of doctors who'd treated them with surgery, x-ray
and radium and finally had given them up as hopeless;
they told how they had come to the Hoxsey Clinic and been
cured. Some of them had been discharged as long ago as
12 years, and showed no signs of malignancy. To support their testimony we put into the record biopsy reports, hospital records, case histories, x-ray negatives and
before-and-after photographs.

We'd subpoenaed three prominent pathologists—Dr.
May Owen, Dr. Marvin Bell and Dr. John L. Goforth—all
good members of the AMA. They testified reluctantly
that they'd analyzed tissue taken from many of those
witnesses, and that it was definitely malignant.

The defense in turn put on a great number of doctors
to testify that the ingredients of the Hoxsey treatment,
individually and collectively, were "*worthless*" and had
no effect whatsoever on cancer. On cross-examination

each was forced to admit that he himself had never tested our treatment on patients, that his testimony was based on theory and not on practical tests.

To rebut the testimony of cured patients, Hearst's attorneys brought in some of the doctors who'd previously treated the witnesses. In some instances these physicians flatly denied any diagnosis of cancer. In cases where biopsies were in evidence, they solemnly asserted that in taking a sample of diseased tissue they'd removed the entire malignancy. In cases where the patient had undergone x-ray or radium before coming to us, they calmly affirmed that those treatments were responsible for the victim's ultimate recovery. And when no other explanation occurred to them, they ascribed the patient's amazing recovery to "spontaneous recession." The organism had healed itself.

According to these doctors, all our witnesses fell into one of three categories:

1—They never had cancer;

2—They were cured by conventional treatments;

3—They cured themselves.

Confronted in cross-examination with obvious discrepancies in their testimony, the sage scientists squirmed and stuttered, twisted and dodged.

If there was no diagnosis of cancer, why did the patient and his family testify in this court that his doctor told him he had cancer? They were *"mistaken!"*

If the entire malignancy had been cut out in the course of biopsy, why did the doctor recommend further surgery? *"No such recommendation!"*

If the patient had been cured by x-ray or radium, why did he still display large nodes and other symptoms when he came to us? *"Delayed action";* the beneficial results of approved treatments are not always immediately apparent.

How many cases of spontaneous recession are known to medical history? *"Quite a few"*—well, maybe one in 100,000 cases.

Such evasive, far-fetched and illogical replies contrasted very poorly with the simple, direct conviction of patients who'd testified that we'd cured them of cancer. The defense would have to do better than this to discredit the Hoxsey treatment and justify the libels.

The very able Hearst lawyers knew this, and had an ace in reserve. Suddenly they produced it: the alleged death certificate of my father, which they offered in evidence. We were amazed. Since 1926 my attorneys had searched high and low through town, county and state records, and failed to find it. It had disappeared from the files shortly after the AMA first sent its agents into Illinois to investigate me.

Examining the document, I immediately spotted it as a phony. It had been filed Jan. 2, 1926—almost 7 years after Dad's death! It stated that he died of cancer! It said he was buried at Girard, Ill. (he actually was buried in the Hoxsey family cemetery in Bond County, more than 60 miles away). And it lacked the signature of the attending doctor! (Dr. Britten, who signed the original, was dead.)

Accompanying it was an affidavit from the widow of a Girard doctor (he'd died in 1923) stating that her husband had told her that Dr. Britten had told him that my father had died of cancer.

It was a foul blow, and it caught us off balance. We

vigorously protested the admission of these two documents as evidence. The purported death certificate was a brazen forgery; and the affidavit, even at face value, was third-hand evidence. But Judge Atwell overruled us and let them go into the record.

The defense had another surprise for us, but this time we were forewarned. We'd gotten a flash over the grapevine that Dr. Fishbein had slipped into Dallas and was hiding in the courthouse library, waiting to testify as a "surprise" witness.

So we were well prepared when a pompous, florid, heavy-set little man with a bald head fringed in greying hair, shrewd eyes behind horn-rimmed spectacles, and heavy jowls emphasized by "5 o'clock shadow," took the stand. He looked like what he was—95 percent politician and publicist, 5 percent doctor. He'd been called in to put the official AMA Seal of Acceptance upon the accusations against me, and he performed his job with obvious relish and full appreciation of his own importance.

He took full responsibility for the *American Weekly* article:

"The article was prepared by assembling material from the (AMA) Bureau of Information, going over the material with Mr. Engle. Mr. Engle then prepared a draft which I then revised and reworked and sent back to him. He then revised and reworked it, then I reworked the final draft."

He declared he was not motivated by "any personal animosity or feeling against Harry M. Hoxsey as an individual." Asked what did motivate him in writing the article, he began to lecture:

"The purpose is the exposé of fraudulent medicine for

the protection of the public, and that has been routine practice, in accordance with the principles and ethics of the AMA ever since it was founded in 1840 . . ."

The Court, which several times had found it necessary to admonish the same witness to confine his answers to a simple "yes" or "no," broke in impatiently:

"No, never mind that. Answer the question. Why did you do it?"

Fishbein, somewhat deflated, replied: "It is part of a practice that has been going on many years."

On cross-examination he admitted that he'd never practiced medicine in his life, nor treated any patients.

He admitted he'd never administered the Hoxsey treatment or any other treatment for cancer, yet insisted he was an authority on the disease.

Asked if his investigators had lifted my father's original death certificate from official files and caused a new one to be made, his reply was: "Not to my knowledge." He said information that Dad had died of cancer first came to him "in letters from physicians in Taylorville, Ill., somewhere around 1926 and 1927."

Asked to identify the "eminent Jurists" hoodwinked and deceived by Hoxsey, he came up with the name of Sen. Elmer Thomas. Counsel reminded him that the Senator never held a judicial position, and the word "*jurists*" was plural, but the witness blandly denied the implication that Texas judges had been hoodwinked by Hoxsey. As for "other important persons" deceived, he said he meant members of the Oklahoma State Legislature.

As the questioning turned to the part he played in persecuting me through the years, he frequently sought refuge in "I don't remember," "I have no memory of it," etc. When he couldn't remember whether his office had sent telegrams to the Legislature in an effort to halt its investigation of Hoxsey, nor whether it had mailed out reprints of the *American Weekly*—both events within the past two years—even the judge registered disbelief.

In fact we didn't press the cross-examination as far as we might have. We had other plans for him. When court recessed he was accosted by a process server who slapped a summons on him. As soon as I learned he was in town I'd filed a libel suit against him in the State District Court. This time he wasn't going to evade service.

Argument in the Hearst case ended on March 18th, and that same evening Judge Atwell rendered an oral opinion.

He carefully avoided passing judgment on the merits of the Hoxsey method, but he indicated clearly that it could not be dismissed as mere "quackery":

"There are 57 people who have taken this stand and said they had cancer. It must be granted they are not learned diagnosticians. Some of them had been treated for cancer before by those who were learned in that particular profession, and their ailment was pronounced cancer. They testified they went out here to the Plaintiff's place and were healed, made well. Defendant wanted the Court to not permit that testimony. I could not do that, and it is in here and must be considered. There is not any way to get away from it.

"So I wish to say, pay your money and take your choice. Those who need a doctor, if you think one side is the best, go and get him. If you think the other side is best, you certainly have the right to go and get him. This is a free country, that is what we stand for in America."

He found as a fact that the article in question did contain libel and slander. He found that its publication did not damage me except nominally, did not cause any substantial decrease in my earnings. And he found that the publisher was not motivated by malice, but by "a mistaken sense of public duty."

Therefore he awarded me token damages of one dollar, and another dollar on behalf of my dead father. Court costs against defendant.

It was not the clear-cut victory I'd expected, but I was satisfied. Fishbein and the AMA were my real target, not Hearst. And this trial had made it possible for me to bring the others into the public arena for a real showdown soon.

For three years, by one legal maneuver or another, Fishbein managed to put off the day of reckoning. His lawyers went from court to court, filed every conceivable motion to dismiss.

They petitioned that the case be tried in Chicago because the defendant lived there, and were denied. They moved to get it transferred to the Federal Courts, but discovered that we'd anticipated them there. (In Texas a State District Court has jurisdiction if any one of the defendants resides in that District, and we'd amended our complaint to include as co-defendant Millard Heath, secretary of the Dallas County Medical Association.) They applied to the Fifth Court of Civil Appeals for a severance and change of venue, were denied, appealed to the State Supreme Court in Austin and were turned down again. Never in the history of Texas has any defendant in any suit—civil or criminal—fought so hard to avoid trial.

What was Fishbein afraid of? For 25 years he'd said he had ample proof that I was a "quack and charlatan." One would think he'd be willing and anxious to expose me in open court!

The fact is, a few months after his appearance in the Hearst case Fishbein had been dealt a stunning blow. The little man long regarded by many as Supreme Poobah of American medicine had been summarily and ignominiously fired by the very organization he'd ruled for 25 years. (See Chapter 8.)

Now when he appeared in court he no longer had the protection of the mantle of authority he'd once worn as acknowledged spokesman for organized medicine. He was merely Morris Fishbein, M.D., a private citizen accused of slandering another private citizen, Harry M. Hoxsey.

That's why he postponed the evil day as long as he could.

Hoxsey vs. Fishbein was scheduled for trial on April 7, 1952. Two days before that date defendant's local attorney, Richard Scurry, came to my office and urged me to agree to a continuance. He suggested that a settlement out of court might be arranged. I advised him I wasn't interested in any settlement, I wanted to prove in open court that the charges his client had broadcast for more than 25 years were vicious lies. Furthermore I'd already issued subpoenas to 300 witnesses in various parts of the country, and it was too late to recall them.

Scurry begged and pleaded, and finally I told him I'd agree to a continuance on one condition: he must go before the judge and promise that his client would either appear for trial on a stipulated date, or publicly confess judgment and pay full damages. He accepted, and we arranged the continuance.

The chips were down now. Fishbein had to fight, or surrender unconditionally. He elected to fight.

The battle began on July 14, 1952, before Judge W. L. Thornton—the same jurist who'd presided when Richards unsuccessfully sued me for damages—and a jury. Again, as in the Hearst suit, the crucial issue was the effectiveness of the Hoxsey treatment. And the evidence followed substantially the same pattern as before.

A parade of former patients took the stand to testify that we'd cured them of cancer. The defense countered with a procession of eminent doctors who swore that our treatment was "worthless." This time the AMA had rallied the cream of the profession; its witnesses were connected with Johns Hopkins, the Mayo Clinic and other top-flight institutions specializing in cancer and cancer research.

One significant episode occurred early in the trial. We had put on several external cases, and my lawyer Herbert Hyde was about to question another one, when defense counsel stood up and declared:

"All right, Herbert, we'll admit you can cure external cancer. We're not arguing about external cases, it's internal we're interested in!"

It was a tremendous concession. For years Fishbein and the AMA had insisted that my treatment wouldn't even cure warts. Now they publicly admitted that we cured external cancer. But it was too little and too late. Before we were through, we intended to prove that we cured internal cancer as well.

This time when Fishbein took the stand we went after

him hammer and tongs. We turned the spotlight on his scholastic pretensions, made him confess that he was unable to get a passing grade in anatomy in his final exams. We forced him to admit that although he never completed his interneship, practiced medicine or treated a single patient in all his life, he had amassed a small fortune advising millions of Americans *"What to Do Until the Doctor Comes."* Before he got off the witness stand he was sweating blood.

And this time the defense made no attempt to introduce into evidence the fake death certificate of my father. Fishbein's counsel knew we could rebut it and prove its fraudulence in detail and in whole. We had witnesses who were present when the original was signed and would testify that the cause of death was listed as erysipelas. We had affidavits and letters from local lawyers to prove that the real certificates had been lifted from the official files. And we had a burial certificate and cemetery records to prove that Dad actually was buried in Bond County, not in Girard as alleged on the fake.

The trial lasted more than three weeks. At its conclusion Judge Thornton handed the jury 34 special issues to decide.

And the jury decided every one in my favor!

It ruled that the preponderance of evidence indicated that practically every phrase referring to me in the American Weekly article was false and tended "to injure the reputation of the plaintiff," impeach my "honesty, integrity and virtue" and expose me to "public hatred, contempt, ridicule or financial injury."

It ruled that the sentence *"Hoxsey has had more than 20 years in which to prove such virtues as might have ex-*

isted in his method" was false. And that the next sentence, *"Such proof has never been forthcoming"* was also false.

It ruled that the phrase *"diagnosis has never been made by scientific methods"* was false.

It ruled that I did not hoodwink and deceive *"eminent Jurists and other important persons."*

It ruled that the article was not written "in good faith, upon reasonable grounds for believing the matters stated therein to be true." And it found that Fishbein had "acted with malice in doing the things inquired about."

However it found that I had sustained no actual damage "directly and proximately" as the result of the article, and so it fixed no monetary award.

In his written decision, Judge Thornton declared:

"This is the second jury of twelve (12) men that has found in my Court that the Hoxsey treatment cures cancer, I have sat here and listened to over fifty (50) witnesses from all walks of life who say that they have been cured. They have showed their scars; they have given the names of the doctors that operated on them or treated them with x-ray or radium. I have heard the testimony of prominent and eminent pathologists, some of whom I know personally, saying that these patients were suffering from cancer before they went to Hoxsey.

"I am of the firm opinion and belief that Hoxsey has cured these people of cancer. And the fact that this jury has answered all questions proves that Hoxsey has been done a great injustice and that the articles and utterances by defendant Morris Fishbein were false, slanderous and libelous.

"Therefore, I am going to award a judgment in excess of one dollar ($1.00) and will make the total judgment one dollar and five cents ($1.05) and assess all costs to the defendant. I feel that this will give Hoxsey a clear vindication, which I know he was seeking far more than he was a money judgment."

In newspaper interviews before this trial Morris Fishbein had boasted: "I have been sued altogether for a total of $30 million. I never have lost a case or settled a case out of court."

Well, he lost this one!

The Government Takes a Hand

In 1950, following my victory in the Hearst case, I made another attempt to get the National Cancer Institute to investigate the Hoxsey treatment. Three years before the National Advisory Cancer Council had fixed three conditions which had to be met before it would consider investigation of any new cancer treatment. On June 6th I submitted 77 case histories, and in a covering letter to Dr. J. R. Heller, Director of the NCI, indicated my belief that they complied with the Council's requirements, as follows:

"1—The method of treatment must be explained fully. There must be no secrecy whatsoever in regard to the composition or the nature of the treatment."

I enclosed a copy of all our formulas, together with a full description of the treatment.

"2—Complete clinical records must be submitted of a suitable number of cancer patients, treated with the remedy or method in question under competent medical supervision, and in each such case the diagnosis of cancer must rest on competent and verifiable microscopic examination."

A minimum of 50 cases was required; we submitted 77. Each was fully documented with clinical records and pathological reports. Some were accompanied by the actual microscopic biopsy slide; where this was lacking the name of the doctor, hospital or pathological laboratory where the slide could be obtained was indicated.

> "3—The records must show that the patients survived at least 5 years following treatment."

All but a few of the cases we sent in had been cured more than five years, and those few were of a deadly type of cancer where survival for even three years was considered little short of miraculous.

About a month later I received a letter from Dr. Heller stating that the NCI could not undertake an investigation of the Hoxsey treatment because of specified deficiencies in the material submitted. My staff put in six weeks of hard work to provide him with additional material, and I sent it on with a letter assuring him that I would leave no stone unturned to comply fully with the requirements of the NCI.

It was a waste of time. On Nov. 1, 1950 Dr. Heller wrote me as follows:

> "This will notify you that the National Advisory Cancer Council on October 29, 1950 reported that it had considered the records submitted in support of your request that methods of cancer treatment of the Hoxsey Cancer Clinic be investigated by the National Cancer Institute.
>
> "The Council concluded that these records did not meet the requirements previously established by the Council which must be met by persons or institutions requesting the investigation of new or unusual treatments for cancer.
>
> "With this adverse report of the Council, the National Cancer Institute has also closed its consideration of your request. Records and other data which you submitted in support of your request will be returned under separate cover."

It is a matter of court record that Dr. Heller and the NCI made no effort whatsoever to verify our cases by getting in touch with the patient concerned, the doctor who'd previously treated him or the pathologist who'd made the biopsy report. It is also a matter of record, as we shall soon see, that the NCI had received direct orders *not* to verify these cases.

Instead of scientific investigation, the U.S. Public Health Service had decided upon legal prosecution. As the FitzGerald report (see Chapter 18) points out:

"In fact every effort was made to avoid and evade the investigation by the Surgeon General's office . . . The record in the Federal Court discloses that this agency of the Federal Government (the NCI) took sides and sought in every way to hinder, suppress and restrict this institution (the Hoxsey Cancer Clinic) in their treatment of cancer."

On Nov. 15, 1950 a complaint was filed charging me with violating the Federal Food, Drug and Cosmetic Act by the "false and misleading" labeling of medicine shipped to doctors and patients in interstate commerce.

The charge against me had nothing to do with the labels on the bottles of medicine we shipped, it was based on two pamphlets we mailed out in reply to inquiries, explaining the Hoxsey treatment, detailing some of the cases we'd treated successfully, listing the names and addresses of other patients who'd taken our treatment, and citing testimony presented before Sen. Thomas and in various courts. The Government charged that in these pamphlets our medicines were "falsely represented as effective cures for cancer."

The USPHS told newspapermen that this was not an attempt to put Hoxsey out of business. Perish the thought! The agency didn't have the authority to put anyone out of business. All it was seeking was an injunction prohibiting us from shipping *"mislabeled"* medicine across State lines.

The real purpose and ultimate objective of this move, as we shall soon see, was to pave the way for action in State and County Courts to close down the Hoxsey Clinic, make it illegal for us to treat anyone in Texas as well as in other States, in short to put us out of business and suppress our treatment.

Aware that we were fighting for our very existence now, we hurriedly prepared for battle. We had little time; the case was rushed through with indecent haste.

The trial began on Nov. 15, 1950, just a month after the complaint was filed. The scene was the U.S. District Court for Northern Texas, at Dallas—the same court where the Hearst suit was tried. And the presiding jurist was the same: Judge William H. Atwell. Except that this time he would not be able to avoid passing judgment on the efficacy of the Hoxsey treatment; it was the crux of the issue; on it the Government case must stand or fall.

In view of the importance of his decision, let's take a closer look at this judge.

At the age of 81 William Hawley Atwell was the oldest jurist on the Federal bench. Nearly 10 years before he could have retired on full pay; he chose to remain on the bench because he loved the law. His record was exceptionally good: only two reversals in 27 years. His courtroom manner was incisive, pithy, often abrupt, sometimes wrily humorous. He often cut off witnesses with "Enough of that. Keep to the point!" He was patient but firm with lawyers. "Counselor," he would chide, "won't you please mind the repetition and irrelevance? Kindly hold yourself to the rules of evidence. Surely you know them as well as I." And he never delayed decision. Usually—as in the Hearst case—he handed it down impromptu, as soon as the trial closed. In his chambers hung the dictum: *"Delayed justice is injustice."*

The roster of expert witnesses who took the stand for the prosecution in this case reads like a *"Who's Who in American Medicine."*

There were experts in pharmacology and experimental therapeutics like Dr. David I. Macht of Johns Hopkins and Dr. Max A. Goldzieher of New York, who testified that the ingredients of the Hoxsey medicines "alone and in combination have no effect in eliminating or retarding the growth of cancerous cells." On the contrary, they declared, potassium iodide (one of the basic ingredients of our internal medicine) "increases rather than retards the growth of cancerous cells."

There were eminent cancerologists like Dr. R. L. Clark, professor at the University of Texas Medical School and director of a hospital for cancer research, who testified that the only definite diagnosis for cancer is by biopsy, and the only proper methods for treating cancer are surgery or irradiation. No medicine taken orally, they declared, can cure cancer.

There were distinguished research experimentalists like Dr. William S. Murray, of the Roscoe B. Jackson Memorial Laboratories of Maine, and Dr. George B. Mider, of Rochester, New York, who testified that they'd conducted experiments with the Hoxsey medicines. Five groups of mice were treated with the remedies, and "no beneficial therapeutic effects" on the cancers in the afflicted animals had been observed.

There were ranking Government officials like Dr. Gilcin Meadows, Chief of Technical Services of the NCI, who testified that the Council had turned down our two requests for investigation because "none of the cases submitted met the basic scientific requirements" set by that group.

In cross-examining these "experts" we managed to get in a number of good, hard licks. All but one were forced to admit they themselves had never treated a single case of human cancer, nor examined any patient taking the Hoxsey treatment. And they were forced to contradict or substantially qualify many damaging statements in their previous testimony.

Dr. Macht, who said he didn't treat cancer because "I know my limitations," admitted that potassium iodide "may have some legitimate and useful therapeutic uses."

Dr. Goldzieher stated frankly: "I am not a cancer man." His experience with potassium was confined to animal experiments. And he'd never tried potassium iodide in these; the only form of that chemical he'd actually used was potassium citrate. He admitted that potassium iodide in the hands of a "skilled" person, and with "other combinations," might be beneficial in certain cases. Even more significant, he confessed that some medicines are very effective when used by some doctors, and not at all effective when used by others.

Dr. Clark admitted, on second thought, that he did know of some cases where medicine taken orally had caused "regression and suspension of growth" of the

cancerous tissue, although he "knew" of no cures. He acknowledged that radioactive iodine had been used for
12 to 15 years in the treatment of cancer. And he confirmed the fact that the only way any medication can be
fairly judged is "by seeing its effects on the individual."

Dr. Murray was mouse-trapped into an admission that
he was not an expert in the treatment of cancer, but only
on its behavior. It turned out that the dosage of our
medicine administered to the mice in his experiment had
been determined arbitrarily by Government pharmacolo-
gists. He'd made no blood count or urine analysis, given
the diseased rodents none of the supportive treatment we
give patients. In other words, the entire experiment was
conducted under ideal conditions calculated to disprove
what the USPHS wanted disproved!

Dr. Mider conceded that animal experiments were a
faulty yardstick, at best: "The data obtained from the
study of experiment cancer lesions cannot be applied
directly to the clinical situation." Furthermore, he said that
substances having a beneficial effect on human cancer
often fail to help animal cancer.

From Dr. Meadows we drew the real reason why the
case histories we'd submitted failed to meet the NCI's
"basic scientific requirements":

Q. "Doctor, did you not agree that you would write to all
the doctors of the 77 cases that we submitted to you, to
verify the information that we had furnished, together
with the biopsies we had furnished you?"

A. "I discussed that, Dr. Heller and I both discussed that
possibility. . . . And we also discussed other forms of
investigation. But the Council asked that we not submit
anything to them except what Mr. Hoxsey sent in, and

asked that we not undertake any investigation unless they so recommend. . . ."

Q. "All right, why didn't you write the doctors?"

A. "We didn't write the doctors because that would be an investigation. . . . And we are not undertaking an investigation unless so indicated by the Council."

The principal witness introduced by the prosecution to prove interstate shipment of our medicines, Dr. Lynwood E. Downs of Denver, Colorado, was sympathetic to the defense. He told how he came to our clinic and studied our methods for 6 to 8 weeks. In that time, he said, he observed the treatment of hundreds of patients with cancers of various types. Many of them visibly improved under our treatment. Returning home, he used the same treatment on his own cancer patients. "The results in many cases were moderately good to quite good," he declared.

To clinch the charge that the Hoxsey treatment is ineffectual, the prosecution presented 16 carefully-selected cases from our files. Four of these patients, it was alleged, did not even have cancer when we treated them. Here is the essential trial evidence in these four cases:

Jack T. Davis of Osceola, Ark. In May 1948 a "wartlike growth" was surgically removed from his tongue. A recognized pathologist then found a "sprig of malignancy" in the excised tissue. The patient came to the Hoxsey clinic, took our treatment, was discharged as cured. Just before this trial—some 2½ years after the original biopsy—another pathologist examined the same slide and declared that the previous report "was an error"; the growth was "non-malignant!"

Mrs. C. A. Gatlin of McLean, Tex. She testified under

oath that Dr. R. D. Gist told her she had cancer of the stomach and urged an operation. He denied this, also under oath. Refusing the operation, she consulted several other doctors and they also (she testified) diagnosed cancer. She estimated she paid them close to $5,000 for cancer treatments before coming to the Hoxsey Clinic. She said we cured her. A year later she again had "pains in the stomach" and returned to Dr. Gist. He operated, and according to his testimony found "peritonitis from a ruptured duodenal ulcer of long standing," there was "no evidence of malignancy." No biopsy was made.

Miss Dorothy Bradberry of Dallas, Tex. In 1945 a small tumor was removed from her breast by Dr. A. R. Thomasson. She testified that he told her it was malignant; a biopsy report declaring it "not malignant" was put in evidence. Some 18 months later there was marked pain and swelling in the same breast. According to testimony by Dr. Ray Thomasson it was due to "mastitis," a non-malignant condition. He administered x-ray, but the swelling and pain persisted. In March 1947 when she came to our clinic there were growths under both arms and nodules in both breasts. We diagnosed cancer with metastasis. She testified that we cured her; all pain and swellings disappeared and have not recurred.

Mrs. A. L. Ebel of Houston, Tex. In 1942 Dr. J. C. Alexander performed a biopsy which disclosed cancer of the bladder. According to his testimony, he removed the entire malignancy. The following year she had severe pain and continuous hemorrhages, consulted Dr. C. M. Crigler. She testified that he told her the cancer had recurred and recommended another operation. He testified there was no evidence of recurrence, the symptoms were caused by "a stricture of the bladder neck." Refusing another operation, she came to the Hoxsey Clinic. She testified that we cured her; the hemorrhages ended, the pain disappeared, and neither has recurred.

So in one case we have a dispute between two recognized pathologists as to analysis of suspect tissue. In another we have a dispute as to diagnosis between a patient who says she paid $5,000 for cancer treatments, and doctors who say she paid it for treating (unsuccessfully) an ulcer! In the third case even if we accept at face value the biopsy report (which case No. 1 demonstrates might well be an "error"), it is not disputed that we cured something—mastitis or metastasis. And in the fourth case even if we accept a diagnosis unsupported by biopsy (which a previous Government witness declared essential for the "definite diagnosis" of cancer), we are left with the unexplained fact that our medicine cured without surgery a serious physiological condition which this same doctor said required surgery.

Such curious and involved evidence would tax the wisdom of a Solomon! Surely, out of the thousands of cases treated at the Hoxsey Clinic, the Government with all its facilities for investigation should be able to come up with more conclusive and damaging "proof" than this!

In the remaining 12 cases presented by the Prosecution, the diagnosis was not questioned. Four of these patients had died of the disease. The others either failed to respond to our treatment, or they abandoned it for surgery and x-ray.

That was the Government's evidence.

The first witness for the defense was Dr. J. B. Durkee, at that time Medical Director of our clinic. He testified that during the previous five years he personally had diagnosed and treated between 5,000 and 6,000 cases of cancer, some successfully and some unsuccessfully. He brought out the fact that recognized pathologists refused to do biopsies for us because of intimidation by the AMA. He described in detail his method of examination, diagnosis and treatment, gave particulars in a number of cases he had treated. He stated that the laboratory at the clinic had been approved by the Government for veteran training. And he put into evidence the statement signed by all patients—*"that the Hoxsey Clinic does not guarantee to cure any ailment or disease"*—as proof that we have never claimed our treatment is a "cure-all" or "sure cure" for cancer.

Dr. E. S. Macauley, who was subpoenaed but not used by the prosecution, testified that he'd studied the Hoxsey treatment for a year at our clinic. Since his return to Jefferson City, Mo., he'd used our medicine in the "successful treatment" of numerous cancer patients. He put many of their names into the record.

Then a procession of former patients filed to the stand to testify that we had cured them of cancer. The Prosecution objected vigorously to such testimony on the grounds that a layman doesn't know if he has cancer and cannot tell if he is cured. Overruling these objections, Judge Atwell declared: "If a man is asked what he had wrong with him, he can answer in this court."

Altogether we presented 22 successful cases, 11 of them external and 11 internal. The Prosecution hammered away at each witness with questions like "How do you know you had cancer? How do you know Hoxsey cured you?" They fired back the names of doctors, dates and other facts.

We backed up their testimony with the testimony of pathologists, with biopsy reports, hospital records, x-ray negatives, photographs and other documentary evidence. The mere fact these patients were still alive, years after we'd discharged them as cured, was eloquent evidence that our treatment is effective.

On Dec. 20, 1950, after six full days of testimony, both sides rested and Judge Atwell took the case under advisement. The following afternoon, in a tensely silent, packed courtroom, he read his *"Findings of Fact and Conclusions of Law"* in the case of the U.S. vs. Harry Hoxsey.

Point by point, they upheld the defense.

He found as fact:

"3. That the respondent's treatment is not injurious. Some it cures and some it does not cure, and some it relieves somewhat. That respondents do not guarantee to cure.

"4. That the statements contained in said labels so pleaded are neither false nor misleading. That if in doubt as to the effectuality of the treatment they take the patient on trial, and frequently without charge to the patient.

"5. That the percentage of efficient and beneficial treatments by respondents is reasonably comparable to the efficiency and success of surgery and radium, and without the physical suffering and dire consequences of radium, if improperly administered, and surgery if not successful in completely removing the entire malignant portion."

And in conclusion he held:

"Nevertheless the facts disclosed by the testimony and found as above, as well as the failure of the Government to successfully carry the burden and show by a preponderance of the testimony the correctness of its charges, merits and must have a refusal of the injunctive relief sought and a dismissal of the bill, and such order and decree is accordingly announced."

All hell broke loose. Newspaper and radio reporters were racing for the telephones; spectators were on their feet clapping and cheering; attorneys, patients and utter strangers were wringing my hand and enthusiastically pounding me on the back. When the Prosecutor got to his feet to file objections and motions Judge Atwell couldn't make out what he was saying, and practically wore out his gavel before he could restore relative quiet.

I was so overcome I could scarcely speak. In years of litigation in more than a score of County, State and Federal courts, this was the hardest legal battle I'd ever fought—and the sweetest and most significant victory that had ever come my way. It was all the more impressive considering the formidable stature and strength of the combination of forces arrayed against us.

Comment on the case by the AMA *Journal* (Jan. 27, 1951) under its new editor was notable for its restraint. The article in its Bureau of Information section was headed simply "COMMENT ON COURT OPINION THAT INTERNAL CANCER CAN BE CURED BY MEDICINE"—a tacit concession that our medicines do cure external cancer. And throughout the article I was politely called "Mr. Hoxsey," a pleasant change from the venomous name-calling that flavored editorials printed during the Fishbein regime.

However the tiger had changed none of its spots, its claws though sheathed were still ominously present. The piece stated:

"Courts ought not to allow lay persons to testify that they have had cancer or any other disease, because they can but relate their beliefs, honest or otherwise, on matters on which they have no actual scientific knowledge."

Not even when these beliefs are based on statements made to them by their own doctors, or on scientific biopsy reports which later turn out to be "in error"?

"Furthermore when such testimony becomes the basis for a judicial opinion that medicines for internal cancer having the ingredients listed above are favorably compared to accepted therapeutic measures in cancer, such decisions can only result in incalculable harm to cancer sufferers. Should patients having cancer which is amenable to accepted therapeutic measures abandon them in favor of an internal medicine, they are losing their lives needlessly."

What about the overwhelming number of cases which (See Chapter 3) are not "amenable to accepted therapeutic measures?" What about the vast number of patients who tried those accepted measures, failed to get relief and were sent home to die?

"The Bureau urges the office of the Attorney General of the U.S. to appeal the denial of injunction vigorously. Public Health in the U.S., particularly as respects the dread disease of cancer, deserves such course of action. There is no known liquid medicine which cures internal cancer."

Public Health in the U.S. deserved another course of action: prompt, scientific investigation of the Hoxsey method and any other treatment which produced evidence that it cured cases of cancer—even external cancer.

All we asked was fair and unbiased investigation. All we got was persecution and prosectuion.

The Attorney-General's office obediently appealed Judge Atwell's decision to the U.S. Circuit Court of Appeals. It is curious how closely the brief it filed coincides with the AMA line set forth in the *Journal* article. The Government urged:

(1) That there was "undisputed proof" of specific charges of misbranding;

(2) That it was "prejudicial error" for the trial court to permit laymen to testify that they had cancer;

(3) That the trial court's findings that the Hoxsey medicines are not falsely represented as cancer cures and that they do cure cancer are "clearly erroneous and should be set aside."

This time there was no rush, it was a full year before the appeal came up for argument. On Nov. 26, 1951, attorneys for both sides appeared before the Fifth U.S. Circuit Court, sitting in Fort Worth. No witnesses were called and no testimony taken; the entire proceedings consisted of legal argument based on the trial record.

The Court withheld any decision for more than eight months—long after every other case submitted that term had been decided. Suddenly on July 31, 1952, while we were in the midst of the libel suit against Fishbein— where the effectiveness of the Hoxsey treatment again was the main issue, and many of the same Government "experts" again appeared against us—the Appeals Court (then in recess for summer vacation) dramatically announced that Judge Atwell's decision had been reversed!

The written opinion closely followed the position taken by the AMA *Journal*. The Appeals Courts ruled that Judge Atwell had committed prejudicial error in admitting the testimony of patients:

". . . when the subject of investigation is the existence of cancer, the personal testimony of the lay sufferer is entitled to no weight, since the overwhelming preponderance of qualified opinion recognizes that not even experts can assuredly diagnose this condition without the aid of biopsy and pathological examination.

"Hearsay evidence of what such a person has been told by a physician is entitled to no greater weight."

It ruled that the only known effective treatments for cancer are surgery and irradiation:

"We recognize as we must that the cause, effect and cure of cancer are so obscure and indefinite that there obtains in the entire subject an area of the unknown.

"It is nevertheless the duty of a Court in making determination of questions of such great public moment as those which now confront us to give weighty consideration to the experience of the past and accepted views and findings of science. . . .

"In this, as in other similar matters, that not all or even very little is known about the subject does not require us to disregard that which is known and established."

It ruled that the Hoxsey medicines were not effective in the treatment of cancer:

"The evidence as a whole does not support the findings of the trial court that 'some it cures, and some it does not cure, and some it relieves somewhat.' "

Accordingly this Court entered an order directing that the judgment be reversed and the case remanded to the District Court "with directions that the trial Court order an injunction to issue as prayed."

It was a devastating blow to us, and an even more ominous blow to scientific progress in the field of medicine. For this decision set a precedent by which "accepted views and findings" of a reactionary medical clique—however mistaken—could be used to prevent the use of unconventional or revolutionary methods to fight any disease which conventional treatment failed to master.

This Appeals Court decision vastly strengthened and gave legal sanction to the AMA's monopoly of medical practice. Its ultimate effect would be to prevent patients from consulting the physicians of their choice and from getting the kind of treatment they want.

In a 3-column article headed "MR. HOXSEY HAS A SET-BACK" the AMA *Journal* jubilantly hailed the new ruling and concluded significantly:

"State authorities in Texas should study this decision. They should consider seriously taking appropriate action to protect the citizens of that state and others who may go to Mr. Hoxsey's 'clinic' in a vain search for a cure for cancer."

Here was a clear statement of the ultimate aim of the prosecution inspired by the AMA and carried out by the Government. Hoxsey must be jailed, his clinic closed, his treatment suppressed!

Government attorneys submitted a proposed injunction decree to Judge Atwell and requested that he sign it, in accordance with the mandate of the superior Court. My attorneys submitted an alternate decree. Both drafts banned the shipment of our medicine in interstate commerce "so long as they are misbranded" by presenting themselves as a cure. The only difference was the addition in our proposal of the words "*without appropriate qualifying statements revealing the conflict of medical opinion as to the truth of such representations.*"

We didn't just pull this phrase out of thin air. When Congress was debating the Federal Food, Drug and Cosmetic Act, many legislators were seriously concerned that this law could be used to prosecute and suppress legitimate medication or treatments opposed by a majority of medical opinion. The intent of Congress was expressed in Report No. 2139 of the House of Representatives, and we quoted this to Judge Atwell:

> "There are clear implications in cases arising under the old Food and Drugs Act and other laws that Congress may not, by a simple and unqualified prohibition against misleading representation, penalize the making of a representation of therapeutic effect regarding the truth of which expert opinion differs. . . ."
>
> "If only a few experts regard a label statement of curative value as true, but the great body of qualified experts in that particular field regard the statement as untrue, there may be substantial ground for concluding that the curative claim is misleading *unless it is qualified in such a way as to show the existence of conflicting opinion as to its truth. . . .*
>
> "The misleading character of the label may be corrected by an appropriate qualifying statement revealing this material fact."

After due deliberation, on June 29, 1953, Judge Atwell approved our draft and signed it as the final decree.

The Government did not appeal that judgment; nor did it file a motion to "alter or amend" that judgment; nor did it move for a new trial. Instead of following traditional procedure, on August 10th it filed an independent action in the Circuit Court of Appeals—an action to which we were not a party, and were not given notice. The complaint declared that the decree did not comply with the mandate of the Appeals Court mandate, which already had ruled that our medicines do not cure cancer, "thus leaving no room for asserted differences of medical opinion." It asked for a writ of mandamus compelling Judge Atwell to strike the qualifying clause from the injunction decree.

For Judge Atwell this was the only time in his long career that anyone had occasion to petition for a writ of mandamus against him. His decision in the Hearst case had been lukewarm, but he was fully convinced his "hot" verdict in the present case was fully justified by the evidence he'd heard. And he was too upright, conscientious and incorruptible a jurist to turn his back on his convictions, however unpopular these might be.

In his reply to the Court of Appeals he wrote:

> "The opinion of this Honorable Court shows distinctly that it recognized there were different opinions as to the curative value and power of the defendant's remedies. . . .
>
> "In addition to such statement by this Honorable Court in its opinion was the great volume of testimony from witnesses in person who appeared and testified that they had been cured of skin cancer by the defendant's treatment and remedies. . . .
>
> "In the oral opinion which I rendered at the conclusion of the trial of the case, I held that the government had not satisfied the burden of proof resting upon it. I still hold that opinion."

On October 22nd the Circuit Court delivered a stinging rebuke to the stubborn Judge:

> "Conceding that the complained of addition to the decree . . . does not conform to the judgment of this Court, he attempts to justify its use in his decree by challenging the correctness of the mandate . . . he asserts in effect

that he has a right to correct our mandate to conform to these views.

"Thus reasserting the correctness of his judgment, which this court has reversed, and the incorrectness of our judgment reversing it, the respondent instead of confessing error in not accepting and giving effect in his decree to the judgment of reversal, defends the reinstatement of his own judgment to the extent accomplished by the addition to the decree. This he may not do."

Under the circumstances there was nothing more Judge Atwell could do. He signed the injunction presented by the Government. Like many doctors, legislators, Government officials and others, he'd learned the hard way that you can't buck organized medicine.

However, in consultation with our lawyers we'd already worked out ways and means to abide by the injunction, and still get our medicine to patients in other states. We discarded the pamphlets which constituted "misbranding"; we stopped shipping medicine to doctors in other states; we made a rule that every patient treated by us would have to be examined by our doctors and given a prescription filled in our laboratory. The label showed only the serial number of the prescription, the name of the patient, the dosage and the signature of the doctor who prescribed it.

My attorneys had written the Food and Drug Administration in Washington to inquire if we could ship medicine so labeled in interstate commerce. In reply we received the following under date of April 23, 1953, signed by George P. Larick, Deputy Commissioner of Food and Drugs:

"You will appreciate that the precise meaning of the phrase 'dispensed on prescription' has not yet been judicially determined. A recent amendment to the Federal Food, Drug and Cosmetic Act . . . requires that certain drugs, including barbiturates, must be 'dispensed on prescription.'

"Your letter indicates that the mailing of the prescribed drug is incidental to the treatment of a patient that the physician has under his professional care. That being the case we would not question that the drug is 'dispensed on prescription' within the meaning of the law."

Under this ruling we continue to ship our medication all over the U.S. to patients who have come to this clinic for examination and treatment. Although the injunction against us is still in force, the Government has not attempted to interfere with any of these shipments.

And despite the injunction, cancer victims continue to flock to us for treatment. No one can prevent former patients from spreading the word that we cure cancer among their neighbors. And whatever the courts may decide as to the legal status of such testimony, the fact remains that it carries far more weight with other victims of the disease than the opinions of all the medical "experts" in the world.

As the eminent Dr. Clark pointed out during the trial, the best test of any treatment is "its effects on the individual."

I am now 54 years young. For 35 of those years I have been kicked, hounded, persecuted and prosecuted because I've treated cancer with medicine and without the use of surgery, x-ray or radium. As the poet says, I've stood "like a beaten anvil" on the theory that the more they beat, the louder the noise; the louder the noise, the bigger the audience; and the bigger the audience, the sooner the truth shall be known.

> " 'How many anvils have you had,' said I,
> 'To wear and batter all these hammers so?'
> 'Just one,' said he; then with a twinkling eye,
> 'The anvil wears out the hammers, you know.' "

"Hoxsey Saved My Life"

ORGANIZED MEDICINE has one infallible formula which it applies to all the evidence we present: *"If Hoxsey cured the patient, he didn't have cancer; if he had cancer, Hoxsey didn't cure him."* Just like the blind man, when he first heard about an elephant: "I wouldn't believe it, even if I saw it!"

Out of the thousands of cured cases in our files I have selected a few to illustrate the different types of cancer we have treated successfully, and the flimsy grounds upon which our claims to cure cancer have been rejected.

All of these are biopsied cases. All of them (with one exception, as noted) have survived and are cancer-free five or more years after they were discharged as cured from our clinic. All of them either were submitted to the National Cancer Institute, or the patient testified in our behalf at court trials or public hearings.

Here is their own testimony, and the evidence to support it. Examine these cases, and decide for yourself if we have reasonable grounds for our claim to cure cancer.

CASE NO. 1—*Frank Anderson, 40, railroad man of Chicago, Ill. Cancer of the lung.*

This is an outstanding case of inoperable lung cancer with diagnosis and biopsy at the Mayo Clinic. Treated by Hoxsey 25 years ago, he is still alive and well, and periodic examinations have disclosed no signs of cancer.

First, his own story:

"In August 1928 I began to get a tickling sensation in my throat. I spit up blood and had difficulty in breathing. My local doctor took x-ray pictures, found a spot on my lung. He could offer no help.

"In April 1930 I went to the Mayo Clinic at Rochester, Minn. I was examined there by a number of doctors, including Dr. Harrington and Dr. Moersch. They found a large tumor in the upper part of my right lung, pressing against the windpipe, told me that I needed an operation.

"The operation was performed by Dr. Harrington on April 16, 1930. He removed one rib and took a sample of the tumor. A few days later he told me and my wife that it was cancer, they could do nothing more for me. On May 5, 1930, I left the hospital and went home.

"About a week later, I heard about Hoxsey, who was in the state of Iowa (Muscatine) at that time. On May 20th I went to see him and began to take his treatment. A month later I stopped spitting up blood and noticed that I could breathe easier. I continued taking his medicine six months more, until discharged as cured.

"I've had no more trouble with my lungs since then. I am a railroad man, have had x-ray pictures taken at 6 months intervals ever since, am working every day. The last x-ray, taken a few months ago, shows no recurrence of cancer."

More than 20 years ago Dr. John H. Lyons of Washington, D.C., became interested in this case and wrote to the Mayo Clinic for information. In reply he received the following letter, dated March 10, 1934 and signed by H. J. Moersch, M.D.:

"Mr. Anderson was a patient here, and there is a very interesting story connected with him. He gave a two-year history of hemoptysis and on examination, a large tumor was found present in the right upper hilus region. I bronchoscoped Mr. Anderson and found the tumor compressing the trachea and made a note that it suggested to me the possibility of an expansile tumor. Dr. Harrington explored him through a transpleural operation and found a very large cyst involving about one-third of the upper right lung. He noted that it was probably filled with blood and degenerating malignant tissue. A specimen was removed, which was examined by Dr. Broders, who felt that the tissue was malignant, but due to the size of the tumor, was unable to definitely grade it.

"I discussed the question of the tumor this morning with Dr. Broders, and he stated that it might be either a squamous-cell, an epithelioma or even a hemangioma, but he could not be certain although he did feel that the tumor was definitely of a malignant nature. Because of this feeling at the time, Dr. Harrington felt that the condition was inoperable.

"I have reviewed the history but can find no evidence of any statement as to his possible duration of life. I am unable to find any record whether Mr. Anderson received any x-ray treatment. However, the gist of the matter is that he was given Hoxley's (sic) treatment, a rather notorious cancer quack, and the last information we received from Mr. Anderson is that he apparently is able to work at the present time and the tumor of the chest has practically disappeared. Dr. Broders informs me that these low-grade epitheliomas sometimes may remain dormant for a long period of time and have been known to retrogress. The situation is a rather difficult one to explain, and the little I know about the matter, I would hesitate very much to try and do so."

In his own subtle fashion Dr. Moersch did try to explain away the fact that we cured Anderson of cancer.

Careful reading of the letter reveals the following contradictions in his explanation:

1—It is stated twice that Dr. Broders "felt" that the tissue was malignant. Cancer cells are visible under the microscope. Dr. Broders is one of the nation's outstanding pathologists. If he "felt" that malignancy was present, he must have found cancer cells in the tissue. Otherwise pathology is not a science, it is a guessing-game.

2—Four years later, informed that the patient had been treated successfully by that *"rather notorious quack Hoxley,"* (sic) Dr. Broders *"could not be certain"* that the tissue actually was malignant, he opined that it might even be a *hemangioma* (a benign tumor made up of newly-formed blood vessels, like a birth-mark)! This afterthought, if taken at face value, must lead to one of two conclusions:

(a) Dr. Broders is not a competent pathologist;

(b) Contrary to the contention of organized medicine and the decision of the Appeals Court, biopsy is not a reliable means of determining cancer.

3—In the first paragraph it is stated that Dr. Broders *"was unable to definitely grade"* the malignancy *"due to the size of the tumor."* In the last paragraph he implies that the malignancy was a *"low-grade epithelioma."* How could he tell if it was Grade I or Grade IV, after this long interval? How could he definitely call it an epithelioma, when in paragraph two it appears that he *"could not be certain"* whether it was squamous cell, epithelioma or hemangioma?

Psychiatrists have a term for this type of rationalization. They call it "retrospective falsification."

To sum up the evidence in the Anderson Case:

1—The patient had cancer. (Established by clinical diagnosis and confirmed by biopsy.)

2—He had no treatment other than the Hoxsey treatment. (Patient's own testimony, Mayo Clinic letter.)

3—He does not have cancer now. (X-ray photos over a period of years.)

No wonder Dr. Moersch found the situation "rather difficult to explain!"

CASE NO. 2—*Mrs. Lora Barnett, 54, housewife of Peniel, Texas. Adeno-carcinoma of the uterus.*

This is a biopsied, 16-year survival case. Yet it is one of those turned down by the National Cancer Institute for lack of *"histological proof."* Here is the patient's own story:

"In July 1939 I began to have severe pains in my lower abdomen and a bad-smelling discharge of blood. About the first of August I went to see Dr. Dickens at Greenville, near my home. He clipped out a piece of tissue and sent it away. About a week or ten days later he notified me that he had gotten back the report and wanted to see me. I went to his office with my husband, and Dr. Dickens showed us the report. It said I had adeno-carcinoma, which he explained was cancer. He said it was very bad, my only hope was radium treatments.

"Two of my friends who had been treated at the Bryan and Peak Cancer Clinic in Dallas told me about the Hoxsey treatment. I was very skeptical, but I didn't know anywhere else to go because I'd never heard of any other doctors that could cure cancer. So on August 16th I went there. Dr. Hartzog examined me and said I had cancer of the uterus. He gave me a bottle of black medicine and a box of brown tablets. I was to take a tablet before each meal and a teaspoon of the medicine afterwards, and come back in a month.

"On my second visit I told Dr. Hartzog I wasn't feeling any better. He said: 'Oh, yes, you'll feel better soon.' And I still did not think that cancer could be cured.

"Well, about six weeks after I started the treatment the discharge stopped, I didn't suffer scarcely any. When I overworked I would feel a little bad, but after 10 or 11 weeks I began to feel like I was well.

"I kept taking the treatment for about six months, then stopped because I was completely well. I haven't had any trouble since. I am now 70 years old, do all my housework and yard work, even make my garden. I don't need any help."

Mrs. Barnett has visited us regularly for examination, and we are unable to find any signs of cancer.

Oddly enough, when we subpoenaed Dr. W. M. Dickens to testify in the Hearst case, he couldn't remember anything at all about Mrs. Barnett. According to the records he brought in he'd examined her only once. He couldn't recall her complaint, didn't remember taking any sample of tissue or receiving a laboratory report. Yet both Mrs. Barnett and her husband testified to these facts.

Moreover the original histopathological report from the Medicolegal Laboratory at Houston, Texas, is in my files. It is dated Aug. 5, 1939, the Lab. No. is 23546. The name of the patient is given as *"Mrs. Barnett"* and it states that she was referred by *"Dr. W. M. Dickens."* (See reproduction on p. 310.) The findings are as follows:

"Section shows irregular acini closely approximated to one another and lined by several layers of columnar epithelium. Stroma shows inflammatory reaction. Conclusion: *Adeno-carcinoma of uterus.*"

The analysis is signed by V. G. Isvekov, M.D., LL.B., Director of the Laboratory.

Yet when the National Cancer Institute wrote to this same laboratory and requested a loan of the slide in this case, it received the laconic reply *"No biopsy under that name"!*

Someone is lying. One way of finding out who it is would be to have a handwriting expert examine Dr. Isvekov's signature on the biopsy report and state whether it is genuine.

The facts in the Barnett case:

1—The patient had cancer. (Biopsy report.)

2—The patient had no treatment other than the Hoxsey treatment. (Her own story, testimony of Dr. Dickens.)

3—The patient is cured. (No recurrence in 16 years following treatment; physical examination discloses no signs of cancer.)

Question: Who cured Mrs. Barnett?

CASE NO. 3—*Clifton H. Smith, 46, flour mill employee of Fort Worth, Texas. Sarcoma, interior gland of neck.*

This is a spectacular 13-year survival case where surgery was impractical and extensive radiation failed to cure. The patient's own story, from a tape recording:

"In July 1939 I began to have trouble with my throat. It felt as if there was something growing inside, on the right side. Then a lump came on my neck just below the right ear. It got bigger and bigger. Within two and a half months it was huge, swelled out like half a football all the way from my ear to my collar bone.

"I went to Dr. Van de Rothgeber who has an eye, ear, nose and throat clinic in the Medical Arts Building, Fort Worth. He thought it was a social disease and sent me to the Terrell Laboratories for a Wasserman blood test. It came back negative. So then he put me in the Methodist Hospital (it's called the Harris Hospital now).

"The next morning he went in my throat with an electric knife. There was a huge mass way back there, and he got a lot of it out, enough to nearly fill a half pint fruit jar. He couldn't get all of it, he said about half the mass was still there and it was wound around my jugular vein, leaving a passage about the thickness of a lead pencil. He called in other doctors to see it. One of them looked at the mess on the table and said: 'My God, what are you doing, taking a woman's ovaries out of this man's throat?'

"They sent the mass to the laboratory, and when the report came back they wouldn't tell me or my wife what the trouble was. All Dr. Van de Rothgeber told her was if I had any business to straighten out I'd better do it because I was hanging on the limb, she was going to be a widow.

"Well, I went back to work and pretty soon a whispering campaign started. One of the doctors who was in on the operation went hunting with a fellow who worked with me and told him that the biopsy had come back cancer. This fellow spread the word at the mill and finally the bookkeeper, who was a friend of mine, heard it. He called up my wife and told her what my trouble was. That's how I found out what was wrong.

"I went to the doctor and asked him what I could do. He said there was but one thing to do, hit it with x-ray or radium. He sent me to Dr. Hyde, an x-ray and radium man in the Medical Arts Building. I went there on Nov. 10, 1939, and Dr. Hyde put on what he called a "block treatment" for about 24 hours. Then he taped five needles to my neck for about five days, eight hours each day. The swelling went away, but I was all red from the tip of my ear down as far as you could see.

"About six months later the swelling came back, two places opened up on the outside of my neck and were discharging pus. I went to the Lisbon Veterans' Hospital at Dallas. Dr. Baker there suggested that the best thing to do was to go to the Hines Cancer Clinic, the Veterans Administration Hospital at Chicago, Ill. So I applied for a reservation. It finally came through, and I went to Hines on Sept. 2, 1940.

"They put me on the table, examined me and found a big mass hanging down like a bunch of blueberries way back in my throat. They went ahead and took another biopsy, and it turned out sarcoma of the interior glands of the neck.

"One of the doctors wanted to take out the soft palate of my mouth, plate it with gold and then give me deep x-ray. But two others advised me not to take the treatment, the mass was too close to the brain, I'd never live through it. I stayed there two weeks, and every night I lay awake and could see nothing but the black box ahead of me. I just made up my mind I wasn't going to take

that deep x-ray. So I refused the treatment, left Hines.
I'd lost 27½ pounds in those two weeks; when I got on the
train I couldn't hardly walk.

"I came back to Fort Worth, and after a while went
to Dr. Hyde and took some more radium treatments, a
series of six settings from Jan. 1941 to April 1941. I was
all burned up, I couldn't take any more. I was a walking
agony, pain and distress. I wanted to die, and I smelled
like I ought to die. The smell was so bad you couldn't
hardly stand it, I was ashamed for anybody to come to
my house. I couldn't talk above a whisper, I couldn't
hardly hear, I couldn't see, I couldn't breathe, I couldn't
sleep. It didn't seem like I could make myself do anything
but stand in front of the mirror and look at my neck,
and see that black box, the wooden overcoat buttoned
up around me.

"Well, one day a friend of mine by the name of Cole
came and told me about the Hoxsey Clinic. So I went
to Dallas. That was on June 8, 1941. Dr. Hartzog was
with Hoxsey then, they both looked me over. They told
me I'd had the infernal Hell burned out of me, there
wasn't but one chance in a thousand they could help
me. I told them I'd take it. 'If you can't help me, put me
out of my misery,' I begged. They gave me a bottle of
black medicine, I was to take it three times a day after
meals and at bedtime. And they told me to come back
in two weeks.

"So help me God, after the fifth dose of that medicine
I waked at two o'clock in the morning and my mouth was
full of blood and I went to the bathroom to dispose of it.
I hung my head over the bowl and suddenly something
popped in the back of my neck, right where my head and

neck join together. My wife woke up and called to me. And I said—just as natural as you please—'I am here in the bathroom.' It like to have scared her to death, my talking like that for the first time in months. She ran in there, then she grabbed the kids and told them. They were sure happy, and I was too. That's the truth, that's exactly what happened, and I'll swear it on a stack of Bibles as high as the tallest building in Dallas.

"My speech came to me, my hearing came back and my eyesight began to get better and better. I kept on taking the medicine for a period of five months. Then the tissue began to break down on the outside, where the radium had scarred it and it had all rotted out. So they put on the yellow powder, they did it twice. It went plumb on through my neck into my mouth and the mass in my throat began to dry up. I guess it was a couple or three months before it came out. The doctor took the forceps, kept working on it from the outside and it all came right on out in a big hard mass with thousands and thousands of little roots. And a piece of my cheek bone came out too, a little snip about the size of a dime.

"I had a hole in my neck. I could take water in my mouth and roll my head to one side and it would run out through the hole, down my neck. It healed and filled in with tissue, now all I have is a little scar on the side of my neck. I began to eat solid food and pick up weight— I weighed only 145 when I first came to the Hoxsey Clinic, and I weighed 189 when I was discharged from there some 18 months later. That was around the end of 1942.

"I haven't had any trouble with my throat since then. I have been examined by—oh, I don't know by how many—doctors. A few years ago I fractured a lobar bone in my back and was laid up in a hospital for a good long while, and doctor after doctor examined me and couldn't find any cancer anywhere."

We have tried several times to get copies of the two biopsies on this patient, but neither the Methodist Hospital at Fort Worth nor the Hines Clinic at Chicago would send them to us. This was one of the cases we submitted to the National Cancer Institute in 1950, and we advised them where the biopsies could be obtained. But they made no effort to do so.

Clifford Smith testified for us in the Government's suit for an injunction against the Hoxsey Cancer Clinic. The Prosecution did not contest the fact that this was a biopsied case of cancer. The only evidence it introduced in this connection was a record of the radium treatments he'd received from Dr. Hyde, laying the groundwork for the contention on appeal that it was radium, and not the Hoxsey treatment, that cured this patient of cancer.

The facts in the C. H. Smith case:

1—The patient had cancer. (Two biopsies.)

2—The patient underwent considerable irradiation, and it failed to alleviate his condition. (His own story, the testimony of his wife and others, physical condition when he came to our clinic.)

3—The patient took the Hoxsey treatment, and has had no other treatment for cancer since then. (Testimony of patient, never challenged in court.)

4—The patient is cured. (No recurrence in 13 years, examination by various doctors shows no cancer.)

Question: What cured Clifton H. Smith?

CASE NO. 4—*Mrs. R. J. Hickman, 51, housewife of Fort Worth, Texas. Melanocarcinoma, anterior left thigh.*

This is one of the most remarkable cases in our files.

Malignant melanomas are the most virulent of all cancers. Arising in cells which produce the pigmentation of the skin (*melanin*), they are the fastest growing of all tumors and have the greatest tendency to metastasize. No neoplasm disseminates more widely or involves more organs. Frequently even before the primary lesion is noticeable, metastases already are so widespread that the case is hopeless.

For that reason cures are rare. According to *Ackerman and Regato,* prognosis is as follows:

"1—Distant metastases when first seen: hopeless, and no treatment indicated. Expected duration of life: one-half to three years.

"2—With clinically obvious positive regional lymph nodes: five year survival, even with lymphatic dissection, less than 5 percent.

"3—Clinically negative nodes proven positive under microscope: prognosis only fair, five year survival probably less than 10 percent.

"4—Lymph nodes clinically and pathologically negative: five year survival 30 percent, with prophylactic regional dissection."

All authorities agree that the prognosis of an actively growing malignant melanoma is unfavorable.

As for treatment, x-ray and radium are of no use since malignant melanomas are radio-resistant. Surgery is the recommended procedure, with wide excision of regional lymph nodes since it is there that metastasis first occurs. A number of eminent cancerologists (among them Drs. George T. Pack, I. M. Scharnagel and de T.

Cholnoky) recommend amputation of fingers, toes, hands, feet and even more radical amputation of entire legs and arms if metastasis to auxiliary lymph glands is established.

That's why this biopsied, 10-year survival case of malignant melanoma with wide-spread metastases is noteworthy. Here is the patient's own story:

"From birth I had a little dark brown birthmark mole on my left thigh, just above the knee. About 1934 I noticed it was getting darker and growing bigger. Ten years later it suddenly began to itch and burn; I would wake up at night clawing at it. It got to where it was kind of a seed wart, about the size of a quarter and the center, which used to be flat, became jagged-looking. It was giving me misery and pain, I was awfully nervous and lost weight—more than 20 lbs.

"On Oct. 3, 1944 I went to my husband's doctor, Dr. C. F. Hayes, on the North Side. He took one look at the mole and sent me to Dr. Porter Brown, a skin specialist in the Medical Arts Building. Dr. Brown put me on the operating table, went around this place with needles to deaden it, I guess, and cut a small piece out. He put it in a little vial and sent it to Terrell's Laboratory, in the same building.

The next evening my husband and I went back to Dr. Porter Brown's office, and he told us the report had come back melanocarcinoma. He said it was the worst kind of cancer there is, grows like wildfire. He looked at my thigh again, poked at a hard lump in my groin and told me I had to go to the hospital right away, there was no time to lose. He said they'd have to scrape this place on my thigh clean to the bone, and if that didn't do any good they'd have to take my leg off at the hip.

"I told him I wasn't going, because I always heard not to cut on cancer. He said: 'If you don't go you won't be here 30 days from now.' I didn't know what to do, but I knew I wasn't going to let them take my leg off. So I told him not to bother making a reservation at the hospital for me, and had my husband take me home.

"My husband is a barber. The next day he was shaving a man named Smith who works at the Universal Mills, and noticed a scar on his neck, and asked what that was. He said it was a cancer, but it was cured now. (See Case No. 3.) Mr. Hickman said to him: 'My wife has one.' Then this fellow Smith told him about Hoxsey's Clinic in Dallas. He said: 'Whatever you do, take her there.' My husband came home and told me.

"The next morning, October 7th, I went to the clinic. By this time my leg hurt so bad I couldn't walk; my sisters went with me, they had to practically carry me in. Dr. Johnson and a nurse examined me. The place on my thigh was about the size of a tea cup, it was red and angry looking, there was a big black knob in the center of it and water running out of it. The swelling in my groin was about the size of an egg, there were hard kernels under my arm and my breast, you could feel a lump on the side of my neck.

"They said it looked pretty bad, they didn't give me much chance. But they said they'd try to help me. I would take the treatment for six weeks. If I felt better, I could continue it; if not, I could give it up. I told them the way I felt, I didn't have anything to lose.

"They put me on the internal treatment right away,

and about three weeks later gave me the first external treatment. I came back to the clinic every week for 28 weeks. I didn't have to go that often, I just wanted to. Because I knew I was going to get well. Even though my neck swelled to half again its size, and my thigh itched and burned like to drive me mad.

"In January 1945 the swellings started to go down, the mass on my thigh dried up and shrank. In February the whole mass came out in one piece. It was as hard and black as the sole of a shoe. Dr. Johnson asked me if I didn't want to put it in alcohol and show it to my sons. I said, 'No, I don't want the stinky old thing. Just throw it in the waste basket.' It left quite a hole in my thigh, but by May this had filled perfectly level with clean tissue. The lumps in my groin and neck and under my arm and breast had disappeared, I was well. But I continued on the treatment until the end of June, when they told me I was cured.

"That was more than 10 years ago. I'm a widow now, live alone and do every bit of work around the house, including the washing. I come back to the clinic every now and then for a check-up, and to consult the doctors for minor ailments. But I've had no trouble since I was cured."

This, substantially, is the story Mrs. Hickman has told as a Hoxsey witness in three trials—the Hearst, Fishbein and Government suits.

There can be no doubt that Mrs. Hickman is a cured malignant melanoma case. We have a photostat of the original biopsy report from Terrell's Laboratories, signed by Dr. May Owen. The date is Oct. 3, 1944, the Lab. No. 322426. (See reproduction on p. 308.)

We subpoenaed Dr. Porter Brown in the Hearst case. He testified that he'd removed the entire melanoma from Mrs. Hickman's thigh, together with a periphery of normal tissue as recommended in all medical texts. He agreed that if metastasis had previously occurred this operation did not cure the patient. He admitted that he'd seen the mass in the patient's groin the day after the operation, and thereafter recommended that she go to the hospital for a "more radical excision."

In reply to a question by defense counsel as to whether the mass in the groin could have been "postoperative inflammation" and not metastasis, Dr. Brown replied: "*It could.*" It is significant that he did not reply "*It was.*"

The good doctor had maneuvered himself into a very delicate position. If he admitted metastasis to the lymph gland, he was conceding that the Hoxsey treatment cures cancer. If he asserted that the swollen gland was due to postoperative inflammation, he was admitting that he had done a sloppy job and endangered the life of his patient. Besides, how explain away the swollen lymph glands under the arm, the breast and in the neck?

We believe there is convincing evidence that this was a true case of melanoma with widespread metastasis. We believe Dr. Porter Brown thought so too, and that is why he recommended "more radical excision." And we believe the record clearly demonstrates that the Hoxsey treatment cured this patient.

CASE NO. 5—*Mrs. Mildred Rager, 24, housewife of Dallas, Texas. Malignant melanoma of the right leg.*

This is a 7-year survival case of proven malignant melanoma diagnosed and treated exclusively at the Hoxsey

Clinic. The biopsy was performed at this clinic, and the patient received no treatment other than the Hoxsey method. Her own story:

"All my life I had a small mole on the calf of my right leg. It never bothered me until 1947. While shaving my leg with a razor one day I accidentally cut into the mole. Soon after the wound healed I noticed that the mole was becoming darker and increasing in size. It grew to the size of a dime, and began to itch. After a time hard kernels appeared behind the right knee.

"I went to several doctors and they all told me it looked like malignant melanoma. They advised me to have it cut out. Some thought I'd get away with losing only a small piece of flesh, down to the bone; others thought I'd have to lose the whole leg. I was afraid of losing my leg, and wouldn't let them operate.

"A friend told me about the Hoxsey Clinic, said they cured cancer without surgery. She said she had taken the treatment, and been cured. So on Feb. 21, 1948, I came to the Clinic.

"I took the internal medicine about a month, and the kernels behind my knees softened up and disappeared. On March 7th Dr. Durkee (then chief of staff at the Clinic) cut a piece off the sore on my leg and sent it away to a laboratory. At the same time he started me on the external treatment.

"A week later he told me the report had come back, and it definitely said I had a malignant melanoma. He explained that it was a very dangerous kind of cancer, and I'd have to come back every two weeks for treatment and dressing.

"After about three months of treatment the sore on my

leg dried up and was taken out. It left quite a hole there. In July new scar tissue began to form and fill in the area, and the external treatment ended. I continued taking the internal medicine until the end of the year, at which time I was told that I was considered cured, and discharged from the clinic. Now the only sign I ever had cancer is a small scar on my leg."

That was nearly 7 years ago, and there has been no recurrence of malignancy.

We have the biopsy report on Mrs. Rager as sent us by the Stout-Todd Clinical Laboratories at San Antonio, Texas. It is tissue report 15A179, state number 02308, and is signed "B. F. Stout, M.D." The analysis is as follows:

"MICROSCOPIC FINDINGS: Sections show the epidermis to extend downward in long bands. Beneath this there are nests and masses of tumor cells extending to the base of the section. These tumor cells have invaded the epidermis and are composed of cells which show rather marked anaplasia with fairly numerous atypical mitotic figures and with single pycnotic nucleoli. The pigment is seen in only a very few cells. This is a malignant melanoma showing evidence of rapid growth.

"PATHOLOGICAL DIAGNOSIS: Malignant Melanoma."

Mrs. Rager's trouble had been clinically diagnosed nearly a year before she appeared at the clinic. Since the biopsy report specifically indicates "evidence of rapid growth," the nodules behind the knee led us to believe that the melanoma had metastasized into the lymph glands before we treated her.

She received no treatment whatsoever other than the Hoxsey treatment.

Who cured this case of malignant melanoma?

CASE NO. 6—*Richard Metzgar, 16, school boy of Erie,* *Penna. Hodgkins granuloma.*

This is another outstanding case, one of the most impressive cures in our files.

Hodgkins is an advancing fatal disease characterized by enlargement of the lymph nodes. Some authorities consider it an infectious granuloma; however it usually is classified as a malignancy related to the lymphoma group of cancer. According to most medical texts, without treatment death usually results in two to three years. If treated, 20 percent of the cases may survive as long as five years. Rarely do victims survive longer.

Here is a biopsied Hodgkin's Disease case which at this writing has survived 7½ years, and there has been no evidence whatsoever of a recurrence.

First, the patient's own story:

"In August 1946, when I was 16 years old, a lump appeared under my right arm. It became painful, and my parents took me to Dr. Roth in Erie, who treated it with an ointment. It failed to recede and during the following weeks my health began to fail. I lost all desire for food, I just didn't have any energy, I would sleep all the time.

"About the middle of September the lymph glands all over my body began to swell. Some became the size of an ordinary marble, others grew to the size of a walnut. My parents took me to see Dr. Schilling, a prominent physician and surgeon in Erie. After a thorough examination he told my father he was afraid I had Hodgkin's Disease; the only way to be certain was to do a biopsy.

"I was taken to Hamot Hospital in Erie, where a node the size of a walnut was removed from under my right arm. It was analyzed by the pathologist there, and his report confirmed Dr. Schilling's diagnosis. I had Hodgkin's Disease.

"The doctor told my father that no cure for this disease is known to the medical profession. The only treatment is x-ray, which reduces the swellings to some extent and alleviates the soreness. But this treatment offers only temporary relief; in the long run it wouldn't save my life. He also said that nitrogen mustard has been used in some cases, but he did not recommend it because he felt that it might do more harm than good.

"I took one x-ray treatment, lasting three or four minutes. Then my father heard about the Hoxsey Clinic from Tom Chapman of Lawton, Oklahoma, who was visiting one of our neighbors.

"We came to this clinic on Oct. 30, 1946. A number of tests were taken, including blood count and an x-ray photo of my chest, and I was examined by Dr. Durkee. He told my father that the prognosis was poor; so far as he knew, nobody with Hodgkin's Disease survived very long. But he agreed to try.

"We went home and I took the medicine. In about four to six weeks my general condition began to improve, I recovered my appetite and felt much more energetic, the swellings all over my body seemed to be getting smaller and less painful. After about four months of treatment the nodes had practically disappeared and my blood count was up. However I continued taking the treatment until March 1948, when I was discharged by the Hoxsey Clinic as clinically cured.

"That was more than seven years ago. I graduated from high school, took four years of college, enlisted in the U.S. Air Force and served 18 months in Japan with the rating of staff sergeant. I have been examined by several prominent cancer specialists, and of course received numerous physical examinations during my hitch in the Armed Services. None of them were able to detect any trace of Hodgkin's Disease, and there has been no sign whatsoever of any recurrence."

We have a photostatic copy of the original biopsy report on Richard Metzgar by the Hamot Hospital Laboratory (see p. 309).

The facts in the Metzgar case:

1—The patient had Hodgkin's Disease. (Clinical diagnosis, confirmed by pathology.)

2—The patient had one x-ray treatment of brief duration, and it did not cure him. (Medical texts state clearly that x-ray is merely palliative treatment in such cases.)

3—The patient took the Hoxsey treatment.

4—The patient is cured. (Survival more than 7 years, physical examination by numerous civilian and military doctors.)

Ask Richard, or his parents, who cured him!

CASE NO. 7—*John Wayne Seago, age 7 weeks, Rockdale, Texas. Retroperitoneal rhabdomyosarcoma.*

When confronted with irrefutable evidence that a cancer patient was cured by the Hoxsey treatment, and no other reasonable explanation is possible, skeptical doctors frequently ascribe the cure to "faith healing." We convinced the patient he was going to get well, and he got well.

Of course this is nonsense. You can use psychology to stimulate a patient's will to survive, but you can't talk a physical organism like cancer to death; you must kill it by physical means.

And you can't heal a 7-weeks old baby by faith.

That is one of the reasons that the following case is important. We do not maintain that we have cured the Seago baby. This child once had cancer; he took our treatment, and has been discharged as "clinically cured." If there is no recurrence of the disease within the next three years, we shall consider him a positive cure.

Here is the story, as told by the child's mother:

"Our son was born April 14, 1953, by Caesarean section, about 10 days premature. When he was about two weeks old I discovered a small lump in the lower part of his abdomen. When he would cry or stretch his little muscles would contract, and at first I thought it was a muscle. One night a week later when I was changing his diaper I noticed that the lump had grown to the size of an egg. I touched it, and it felt very hard. My husband and I were worried, so next day we took the baby to Dr. Leland Deneson in Cameron, Texas.

"At first he thought it was a hernia; then he felt of it and said it wasn't a hernia because it didn't move. He told us to come back the next day and he'd make some tests to find out if it was a dislocated kidney. He has a clinic, and a lot of doctors from Waco come there on certain days.

"We came back next day and Dr. Martin Even (of Waco) took all kinds of tests and about 7 x-rays. He said it wasn't a dislocated kidney. Dr. Deneson and his nephew, Dr. Marvin Bartlett (the one that did the Caesarean on me) and other doctors there were talking together. Then Dr. Deneson told us he was pretty sure it

was malignant, and if it were his baby it would already
have been taken out.

"We took the infant to St. Edward's Hospital in
Cameron, and he was operated on the next morning,
May 26th. The operation was done by Dr. Bartlett and
Dr. Roy Beskin (of Waco), a surgeon specialist formerly
with the Mayo Clinic. Dr. Deneson came out of the
operating room and told us it looked very bad, there was
a large mass there and it was entwined around the main
artery. I asked did they take it all out, and he said no,
they couldn't cut into it because the slightest slip they
would cut the artery and the child would bleed to death.

"I asked how much they did take out, and he said:
'Just enough to send off to the laboratory.' He said it
looked very much like sarcoma, which is cancer. In fact
they were almost sure of it. He said 'I don't see any
chance for the child.'

"So of course we got frightened and I began to cry.

"What hurt us was that the baby was so tiny and so
small, and he would have to die, and before he died he
would have to suffer so much. You know, that's the way
with cancer. They didn't give us any hope. They didn't
even recommend x-ray or radium. All they said was 'Take
him home, and when he gets bad bring him back and
we'll give him some medicine to ease his pain.'

"Well, my husband called my daddy to tell him about
it, and my daddy had heard about the Hoxsey Cancer
Clinic in Dallas and suggested we find out about it. My
husband said 'If there's any chance whatever I'm going
to take it.' He left for Dallas about midnight. Next day he
saw Dr. Hoxsey, told him about the operation, said we
didn't have much money. Dr. Hoxsey said the money

didn't much matter, if there was anything he could do for the baby he'd be glad to do it, to bring him right on.

"So on June 1st we brought John Wayne to the Hoxsey Clinic. Three doctors there looked at him, gave him blood and urine tests, took x-ray pictures. They said there wasn't much chance, they didn't have much hope because they'd never treated anyone that tiny. (The baby was not quite seven weeks old.) But they said they would try, they'd put him on 60-day trial. They gave us a bottle of the black internal medicine and told us how much to give him.

"We took the baby home and started him on the medicine. The first week we gave him five drops at a time, three times a day. Every week we increased the dose by a drop. By the end of a month, when we took him back to the clinic, he was taking nine drops three times a day.

"Meanwhile we'd taken John Wayne back to the hospital where he'd been operated on, and two doctors looked at him. One of them, Dr. Bartlett said it seemed like the swelling was getting a little bit smaller; the other, Dr. Beskin, said at least it hadn't gotten any bigger. They seemed surprised. We didn't tell them he was on the Hoxsey treatment.

"We took him to the Hoxsey Clinic every month. The second time we were told to give him 15 drops of the medicine three times a day, the third month half a teaspoon after meals, and the fifth month the dose was increased to a full teaspoon. At that time he seemed to be getting along so well that we didn't have to bring him back for three months.

"In September we took John Wayne to Dr. Travis Greene here in Rockville. They seemed to have lost interest in him at Cameron, and besides Dr. Greene was much closer. When he first looked at the child the lump was about the size of a pecan. It was definitely getting smaller. We told him about the Hoxsey Clinic, and he said he didn't blame us for going there; under the circumstances he probably would have done the same thing.

"A few months later when Dr. Greene examined the child he said he couldn't be sure if he felt a knot, but if he did it was about the size of the end of his finger.

"When we brought the baby to Dr. Greene for examination in February, he was amazed. He felt all over the baby's abdomen for the knot, but couldn't find it. It just had disappeared!

"About the end of May they told us at the clinic that they thought the baby was cured, we could take him off the medicine, but to bring him in every six months for examination.

"Our baby is 2½ years old now. He's healthy and normal in every respect; he eats, sleeps and plays like other children; there has been no sign of anything wrong with his abdomen, except the scar of the operation."

We learned that the tissue from the Seago baby was sent to the Scott and White laboratory at Temple, Texas, for analysis and have made several attempts to get copies of it, with no success. The laboratory refuses to release it to any doctor who is not a member of the AMA.

A reporter for a national magazine who investigated this case also tried to see the laboratory report, but had no better luck. He called Dr. Deneson, and the latter refused to talk about the Seago case or to see him. He did talk with Dr. Greene.

Dr. Greene said he happened to be at St. Edward's Hospital the day the baby was operated on. It was such a rare case that a number of outside doctors were invited into the operating room to observe it, he among them. He said he saw a large mass in the baby's abdomen pushing aside the intestines. It appeared to be attached to the vertebra and was wound around the *aorta* (the main artery) and the *vena cava* (a vein carrying blood to the heart). The concensus of medical opinion was that it was malignant and inoperable. He said he'd previously seen two similar cases, both were malignant and both patients eventually died of cancer.

Later, when John Wayne Seago became his patient, Dr. Greene said, he took the trouble to look up the biopsy report. It stated that the specimen submitted was inconclusive (the tissue had deteriorated, probably from faulty solution). However the report stated that from the appearance of the sample as well as the case history "a diagnosis of *retroperitoneal rhabodomyosarcoma* must be assumed."

The prognosis was zero. Yet the child is alive and healthy today. (See photos on p. 150p.)

In April 1954 ten M.D.s from various parts of the country who had come to our clinic to investigate the Hoxsey treatment studied the Seago baby's case history, saw the x-rays, questioned the parents, and examined the child, (he was still under treatment at our clinic). They were unable to find any trace of the swelling, or any evidence of cancer.

We believe the child is cured. We'll *know* he's cured three years from now, if there is no recurrence.

The Fight Continues

THE CASE histories detailed in the previous chapter are typical of those we have submitted over the years in a vain attempt to obtain a fair and impartial investigation of the Hoxsey treatment. Only one conclusion can be drawn from the failure of the AMA to consider seriously the proof that we have offered, or to sanction sincere consideration by some responsible Government agency:

Organized medicine fears that an honest investigation will establish the fact that we cure cancer.

The alarming proportions of the ruthless conspiracy to suppress all unorthodox cancer treatments—regardless of what scientific merit they may have—is revealed in a 1953 report by special counsel to the U.S. Senate Interstate Commerce Committee which may be found in the *Congressional Record* (Aug. 28, 1953, pp. 5690-93).

This report has a fascinating history.

For many years the late Sen. Charles Tobey of New Hampshire—whose son had been cured of lung cancer by unorthodox methods—vigorously fought for a full-scale Congressional investigation of cancer research and treatment in this country. He couldn't get it; every move in that direction was skillfully blocked by the AMA.

Early in 1953, when he became chairman of the Senate Interstate Commerce Committee, the Senator hit upon a clever way around the roadblock. Without telling any of his colleagues he set up a staff to conduct a secret preliminary survey of the cancer situation, with special attention to *"the alleged interstate conspiracy engaged in by any individuals and combines of any kind whatsoever to hinder, suppress or restrict the free flow of drugs, research and methods relating to the cause, prevention and systems of diagnosis and treatment"* of the dread disease. He was confident that the survey would uncover enough dynamite to blast Congress out of its complacency and force it to authorize a full-scale investigation.

Casting around for a capable and energetic individual to head this probe, he consulted his friend U.S. Attorney General Herbert Brownell. The latter recommended a clever, 35-year-old lawyer then employed as trial attorney for the Department of Justice: Benedict F. Fitzgerald, Jr., who previously had served as attorney for the National Labor Relations Board and counsel to a Congressional Committee investigating lobbying activities. Fitzgerald thereupon was directed to finish his work at the Department of Justice and report to the U.S. Senate, on a loan basis, where as special counsel to Tobey's committee he was assigned to the cancer probe.

Within six months Fitzgerald and his aides had uncovered enough sensational evidence to blow the roadblock sky high, if properly triggered. He sat down to write a report on his findings. Unfortunately just before it was finished Sen. Tobey died of a heart ailment (July 24, 1953). He was succeeded by Sen. John Bricker of Ohio. A few weeks later the new chairman received Fitzgerald's report. It was a blistering indictment of the

AMA and its coercive and monopolistic activities in the field of cancer research and treatment.

For example, it revealed that Dr. J. J. Moore, treasurer of the AMA, had offered the discoverers of *krebiozen* $1½ million for exclusive rights to the cancer drug, on behalf of a leading pharmaceutical house. When he was turned down, the AMA began to denounce the drug as "worthless" and to lop off the professional heads of its backers— including Dr. Andrew C. Ivy, then vice-president of the University of Illinois and head of its medical school.

The Fitzgerald report stated:

"There is reason to believe that the AMA has been hasty, capricious, arbitrary and outright dishonest, and of course if the doctrine of *'respondeat superior'* is to be observed, the alleged machinations of Dr. J. J. Moore (for the past 10 years the treasurer of the AMA) could involve the AMA and others in an interstate conspiracy of alarming proportions . . .

"Behind and over all this is the weirdest conglomeration of corrupt motives, intrigue, selfishness, jealousy, obstruction and conspiracy that I have ever seen."

The investigators spent considerable time studying the Hoxsey controversy. Subsequently, in a letter to Sen. William E. Langer, Fitzgerald wrote:

"From the evidence I have gathered, it appears that as early as 1924 the Hoxsey method of treating cancer was considered so effective by a former president of a medical association that he personally presented its sponsor with a written proposal which, among other things, provided for the relinquishment of valuable property rights in the Hoxsey method and medicines and formulas to this same official.

The evidence indicates that when the proposition was spurned, Hoxsey was advised to sign and accept the proposal or face ruination.

"Such tactics, if true, constitute blackmail of the rankest order and this evidence should be examined closely to ascertain its credibility."

He devoted eight pages of his report to cite specific instances of the AMA's struggle to suppress the Hoxsey treatment. Speaking of Sen. Thomas' fruitless efforts to get the Surgeon General to undertake an investigation of our Clinic, he remarked:

"No such investigation was made. In fact every effort was made to avoid and evade the investigation by the Surgeon General's office."

Relating our bitter experiences with the cases we'd submitted to the National Cancer Institute, he declared:

"The record in the Federal Court discloses that this agency of the Federal Government took sides and sought in every way to hinder, suppress and restrict this institution in their treatment of cancer."

The report listed numerous other unorthodox cancer treatments which had experienced similar obstruction by the AMA. Summarizing the evidence, it pointed out the urgency of a full Congressional investigation:

"If neither X-ray, radium or surgery is the complete answer to this dreadful disease, and I submit it is not, then what is the plain duty of society? Should we stand still? Should we sit idly by and count the number of physicians, surgeons and cancerologists who are not only divided but who, because of fear or favor, are forced to line up with the so-called accepted view of the AMA?

"Or should this committee make a full-scale investigation

of the organized effort to hinder, suppress and restrict the free flow of drugs which allegedly have proven successful in cases where clinical records, case histories, pathological reports and X-ray photographic proof, together with the allegedly cured patients, are available?

"Accordingly, we should determine whether existing agencies, both public and private, are engaged and have pursued a policy of harassment, ridicule, slander and libelous attacks on others sincerely engaged in stamping out this curse of mankind. Have medical associations, through their officers, agents, servants and employes engaged in this practice?

"My investigation to date should convince this committee that a conspiracy does exist to stop the free flow and use of drugs in interstate commerce which allegedly have solid therapeutic value. Public and private funds have been thrown around like confetti at a country fair to close up and destroy clinics, hospitals and scientific research laboratories which do not conform to the viewpoint of medical associations.

"How long will the American people take this? . . ."

Sen. Bricker—a sturdy supporter of AMA policies in Congress—took one look at the scorching document, deposited it carefully in a fire-proof wastebasket and promptly put an end to the investigation. He refused to see Fitzgerald, although the investigator offered to fly to Ohio at his own expense for an interview. Instead his office advised the former special counsel to "forget" the whole thing; and above all, *not to talk to the press!* If he played ball, he would *"be taken care of."*

Fitzgerald, a conscientious and brash citizen, refused to play ball. He wrote the Senator a sharp letter in which he said he was "surprised and even shocked" at the runaround, sent copies of the letter and report to every senator on the committee, managed to get the report read into the *Congressional Record*. And there it lies buried.

His job with the committee abruptly terminated, he went back to the Department of Justice, and suddenly discovered that he didn't work there any longer. The AMA had put the finger on him, he was too "hot" to hold down another job in the Government. Now he is engaged in private practice in Washington, getting "hotter" by the minute defending clients who are under attack by organized medicine.

Bricker's loyalty to the AMA was well rewarded. He was guest speaker at the next AMA convention. And soon after that the Association conducted a vigorous campaign on behalf of the Bricker Amendment to limit the treaty-making powers of the President; every doctor in the country got a letter urging him to support the Amendment, medical publications published appeals: "Support the Bricker Amendment!"

This move was severely criticized by many staunch AMA members, who pointed out the obvious: that the Amendment had nothing to do with medical matters, and the Association had no right to throw its weight behind political measures outside the field of medicine. As the eminent Dr. Charles W. Mayo, former alternate U.S. delegate to the United Nations put it, this action *"has the effect of abrogating the right of individual doctors to make up their own mind."*

And that's how the AMA prevented the Government from investigating the conspiracy against independent cancer research and treatment.

We have given up all hope of ever obtaining an investigation. We're not going to plead, beg and challenge any further. We're not going to submit voluminous files of cured cases and other documents hither and yon on the faint chance that some medical group or Government agency will summon the courage to seek the objective truth about our treatment. We're not going to stage any more dramatic demonstrations to prove to the public that we cure cancer.

We know it, our patients know it, doctors, judges and laymen who have gone into all the facts of our long controversy with organized medicine know it. And I sincerely believe that anyone who has read this book through to the end must be convinced that our treatment deserves authoritative consideration.

We shall continue to treat cancer with the Hoxsey method, and defend our right to do so to the bitter end, in and out of court. We shall concentrate on improving that method, and on accumulating scientific data to prove our contention that chemotherapy is the only true effective way to deal with this deadliest of all diseases afflicting modern mankind.

On April 5, 1955, the Hoxsey Cancer Research Foundation was chartered by the State of Texas as a non-profit corporation dedicated to the scientific study of the Hoxsey treatment and its effect on human cancer. Its medical director is Dr. Donald Watt, D.O., whose qualifications include long experience as a research chemist for the Barrett Research Laboratories at Underhill, N.J. The chief laboratory technician is Kenneth Burt, a graduate of the East Texas State Teachers College. He has studied and worked at the Brook Medical Center, San Antonio, where he specialized in blood chemistry.

The recently-installed laboratory of the Foundation

contains the finest and most modern research equipment available today; in setting it up we consciously duplicated the lab equipment of the M. G. Anderson Foundation for Cancer Research and Therapy, widely known as the "Mayo of the South."

The first project of the Foundation is an intensive study of the various ingredients of the medicines used in the Hoxsey treatment, and their effect upon blood serum. Another will be to evaluate the data contained in more than 20,000 case histories now in our files, follow up cases discharged as cured by the clinic and accurately tabulate the exact percentage of successful treatment of various types of cancer. A third will be a study of our basic medication as a possible preventative for this deadly disease.

We sincerely believe that the labors of this Foundation will result in test-tube proof of the efficacy of the Hoxsey treatment, and establish scientifically beyond question or quibble the fact that we cure cancer.

On that we rest our case.

APPENDIX

Reproductions of Letters
and Medical Reports

Evidence of frame-up: letter from [one] of alleged complainants against Hox[sey] in action brought by Texas Board [of] Medical Examiners (Chapter 13). [At] left, papers served on three defenda[nts].

Fee Docket
Book .. .. ..
Page ... .

Judgmen[t]
Book
Page

COUNTY CRIMINAL COURT
Unlawful Practice of Medicine
THE STATE OF TEXAS

vs.

Martha Ho[...]

JAN 5 - 19[...]

Fee Docket
Book ..
Page ..

Judge[...]

COUNTY CRIMIN[AL]
Unlawful Practic[e]
THE STATE OF

Dr. Carrie M. [...]

Fee Docket
Book ..
Page ..

Judgmen[t]
Boo[k]
Pag[e]

COUNTY CRIMINA[L]
Unlawful Practice of [...]
THE STATE OF

vs

Harry M. Ho[...]

Filed   JAN 5 -
Capias Issued   JAN 5 -
Defendant's Att'y H[...]
                    DISPOSITION
FEB 2 - 1937

Dec 30 – 1940

Sweetwater Texas

To the Prosecuting Atty of Dalla[s]
Dallas County Tex.

This is to advise you that I
was never at any time treated
By Harry M Hoxey and at no time
did he ever tell me he was a
Doctor. All the treatments that
I recieved for my condition was
administed by Dr C M Hartzog.
And the state man filed that
case without my consent, and I
will not testify against Mr. Hoxey
for you or anyone else And I urge
you to dismiss this case against
Mr Hoxey as I know it is a frame
By his enemies.   Signed W S Scott

witnessed
Astell Roberts
Jno Fred Slate

302

MARVIN D. BELL, M. D.
CLINICAL PATHOLOGY
1109 MEDICAL ARTS BLDG.
DALLAS, TEXAS

December 5, 1945

Dr. R. R. Braund
U. S. Public Health Service
Baltimore, Maryland

Dear Dr. Braund:

Under separate cover I am mailing you slides which
you requested from patients whom Mr. Hoxsey has claimed
to have cured.

The slide which I find on Mrs. O. G. Brown shows chronic
inflammatory tissue, and I do not know whether I was foolish
enough to call this carcinoma at the time or if possibly
I had another slide which did show carcinoma and was
accidently discarded at the time.

With best regards, I am

Respectfully,

Marvin D. Bell

D. Bell, M. D.

12/12/39

MARVIN D. BELL, M. D.
CLINICAL PATHOLOGY
1109 MEDICAL ARTS BLDG.

Mrs. O. G. Brown   Dr. Hartzog

Sections show a thin layer of surface epithelium
with considerable round cell and plasma cell infiltration in the corium, which is composed of dense
fibrous connective tissue. In the lower portion of
this are a few alveolar collections of round
epithelium with large pecnotic and hyperchromatic
nuclei and a good many mitotic figures.
Diag: Adeno carcinoma in the skin, recurrent,
grade 2.

Marvin D Bell

A pathologist, under pressure, changes his mind. In 1939, he diagnosed cancer. On Dec. 5, 1945, he thinks he made a "foolish" mistake.

303

Texas State Board of Medical Examiners

OFFICE OF SECRETARY

Dallas, Texas

Dec-13-1940

Mr. Jack W. Knight
Investigations Counsel
State Board of Medical Examiners
San Antonio, Texas

Dear Jack:

After reading the attached copy of a report on a recent investigation you will no doubt think I have gone in for a lot of "dusky" business. However it seems that we are having a hard time connecting up a good case on Hoxsey where white people have been treated and the witnesses reside in Dallas County or nearby. This naturally would make it difficult to get the witnesses here for trial.

I am sending this to you for your comment and advice as to whether you think we would stand a chance to stick Hoxsey on evidence which is wholly testified to by negros. It seems that these darkeys all have a clean record behind them and all have been questioned about any previous difficulty with the law and only one has ever been in court and paid a fine. This was Mamie Sneed who paid a one dollar fine in Corporation Court for running a red light on one occassion.

I have another case almost like this one where a negro woman was treated who subsequently died but there is only one witness in this instance. This is her granddaughter. While in this case there are several. What do you think of it?

I have a few other clues and hope by Jan 1st to be able to make a good case involving the treatment of some white person but if we are unable to do it, we would like to start working on him on this case if you think advisable.

It seems that . . . Crowe plans to . . . come up here shortly . . .
. . . forward to seeing you up here soon after the new year. I am

Very sincerely

W. F. McBride

Confidential letter from State Board investigator showing despera[te] attempts to "stick" Hoxsey with conviction on charge of "practici[ng] medicine without a license."

304

United States Senate

COMMITTEE ON APPROPRIATIONS

June 2nd, 1947

Mr. Harry M. Hoxsey,
c/o 4507 Gaston Avenue,
Dallas, 4,
Texas.

Dear Mr. Hoxsey:

I have your favor of May 29th and note the further difficulties you are having in carrying on your work.

It seems that the medical fraternity is highly organized
and that they have decided to crush you and your institution, if at all possible. I have had a few "rounds" with the
heads of the medical organization as well as the Public Health
Service here in Washington and it seems that the public officials are afraid that if they make any move, or say anything
antagonistic to the wishes of the medical organization that
they will be pounced upon and destroyed. In other words, the
public officials seem to be afraid of their jobs and even of
their lives. This presents a most serious case and I am at
a loss to know how to proceed.

I am of the opinion that what the medical organization does
will be repeated by the several state organizations in the
event any Congressman or Senator started out to publicly oppose
their program. I have done what I could to have your remedy
or at least the record of your accomplishments considered and
passed upon but, to date, the authorities here have refused
to act.

If I find wherein I can do anything further to help out I
shall gladly avail myself of the opportunity. If you receive
a reply to your letter to the Pure Food and Drug Administration,
I shall be glad to have a copy of the same.

With all good wishes, I am

                                Sincerely,

                                Elmer Thomas

ET:f

Letter from U. S. Senator Elmer Thomas, explaining his failure to obtain
official investigation of Hoxsey treatment (Chapter 14).

April 29, 1947

Rinaker, Smith & Hebron
Attorneys at Law
Carlinville, Illinois

Gentlemen:

The Department has your letter of April 22
in connection with the matter of the death
certificate of Dr. J. E. Hoxsey, but we
have been unable to find a record of his
death.

We have found a death record for Mrs. Jennie
Hoxsey, who died at Staunton, Macoupin County,
on January 17, 1919. The death record states
that she was a widow, and that being the case
and she was the widow of Dr. Hoxsey, he must
have died prior to 1916.

If you can assist us by supplying more definite
information relative to his death, we will
again attempt to find the record.

We are returning your remittance of $1.00.

By direction of the Director,

Very truly yours,

R. H. Woodruff, M. D.
State Registrar.

RHW:EV
Enc.

Letter from Illinois State Registrar exposing fake "death certificate"
introduced in evidence during Hearst case.

May 25, 1940

Laboratory No. 222894.
Name: Mr. J. A. Johnson, Ranger, Texas
Doctor: J. C. Terrell, Stephenville, Texas
Tissue: From under tongue.

Clinical Opinion:

Findings:

The specimen submitted consists of a small, reddish-pink section of tissue that measure 8 x 5 x 4 mm. One surface is covered with mucous membrane.

Microscopical sections from the small biopsy have a small surface that is covered with a thick layer of well differentiated squamous epithelial cells. A larger surface is covered with squamous epithelium showing a number of bulbous epithelial downgrowths, at the base of which there is a thin layer of loose, vascular, fibrous tissue that contains a few circumscribed groups of squamous epithelial cells. A number of these cells have a large hyperchromatic nuclei and a few show irregular mitoses.

Pathological Opinion: Squamous cell epithelioma, grade 2 (high 2)

TERRELL'S LABORATORIES

BY_____
May Owen, M. D.

The National Cancer Institute found that J. A. Johnson did not have cancer (Chapter 14). Here is the biopsy report: "*Squamous cell epithelioma* (cancer) *grade 2 (high 2).*"

Laboratory No. 322426
Name: Mrs. R. J. Hickman
Doctor: Porter Brown, and C.F.Hayes
Tissue: From leg

Clinical Opinion: Melanocarcinoma

Findings: The specimen submitted consists of four firm
sections of tissue, the largest measures 1.5 x 1 x .8 cm.
A small part of the tumor is pigmented dark brown. The
cut surfaces are firm smooth and pink.

Microsections show the biopsies to be from a melanocarcinoma.
The superficial layers of tissue are very inflammatory and
the ulcerated surfaces of the tumor are covered with inflammatory
exudate. In some areas a thin layer of partly keratinized
epithelial cells covers nests of tumor cells. These epithelial
cells have large vesicular hyperchromatic nuclei and a number
contain large irregular mitotic figures. A number of these
cells contain finely granular brown pigment and in the
connective tissue that supports the groups of tumor cells
there are phagocytic cells filled with a similar pigment.
There are small groups of tumor cells deep in the biopsies.

Pathological Opinion: Melanocarcinoma.

TERRELL'S LABORATORIES

By *May Owen*
May Owen, M.D.

MO/bp

This is the biopsy report on Mrs. R. J. Hickman which the National
Cancer Institute was unable to find. The report's opinion: "Melanocarcinoma." (Mrs. Hickman tells her story in Chapter 17.)

Form A-97-1M-6-45

Hamot Hospital Laboratory

PATHOLOGICAL REPORT

Lab. No.   25073   Date   October 8, 1946

Specimen   AXILLARY GLAND (Right)

Patient's Name   METZGAR, Richard   Age 16

Surgeon's Name Dr. Schilling

Macroscopic Description: Specimen consists of a large irregularly rounded lymph gland from the right axilla. It measures 3.8 cms. in greatest diameter and weighs 10 gms. The lymph gland has been incised. The cut surface of the gland is fairly solid in consistency and yellowish gray in color. No gross areas of necrosis are seen on the cut surface.

Diagnosis: The pathological condition is a rather early Hodgkin's granuloma.

Remarks:

(signature) M. D.
Pathologist

Biopsy report on 16-year-old Richard Metzger shows "*Hodgkin's granuloma.*" Few survive it. Richard is still alive, nine years later. (See his story in Chapter 17.)

MEDICOLEGAL LABORATORY
V. G. ISVEKOV, M. D., LL. B., DIRECTOR
TELEPHONE SADLEY 8102
1400 ELGIN AVENUE
HOUSTON, TEXAS

Lab. No. 23545

AUG 5 1939 ___ 193__

Name ___ MRS BARNETT

Referred by: Dr. _____ WM Drither

MISCELLANEOUS EXAMINATION

Nature of examination: ___ Histopathological

Material: ___ Submitted cervical tissue

Methods used: ___ Paraffin embedding

Findings ___ Section shows irregular acini closely approximated to
one another and lined by several layers of columnar epithelium.
Stroma shows inflammatory reaction.

Conclusion: ___ Adeno carcinoma of uterus

Examined: _____ W. G. Brazel

The National Cancer Institute failed to find a biopsy report on Mrs.
Lora Barnett. Here it is: "*Adeno carcinoma.*" (See her story in Chapter
17.)